WE HAVE MET IN PAST LIVES
A study of past life regression

BRIGITTE CALLOWAY

DHP Acc Hypnotherapist

Copyright © 2019 Brigitte Calloway
All rights reserved. No parts of this publication may be reproduced, stored in a retrieval system or transmitted, in any form, or by any means, without the prior permission of the copyright owner.
A catalog record for this book is available from the National Library of New Zealand.
ISBN: **978-0-473-47833-9**

To Miriam and Amos, forever grateful for your love

CONTENTS

Prologue	1
How we remember past lives	5
Soul groups	15
Karma and karmic lessons	25
Karmic lesson 1: LOVE	31
Karmic lesson 2: SUCCESS	41
Karmic lesson 3: FAMILY	51
Karmic lesson 4: PATIENCE	59
Karmic lesson 5: TRUST	67
Karmic lesson 6: EMPATHY	77
Karmic lesson 7: INTEGRITY	85
Karmic lesson 8: FUN	93
Karmic lesson 9: PROSPERITY	105
Karmic lesson 10: DUTY	117
Karmic lesson 11: KINDNESS	125
Karmic lesson 12: HOPE	131
Karmic lesson 13: SACRIFICE	139
Karmic lesson 14: HARD WORK	147
Karmic lesson 15: CHANGE	153
Karmic lesson 16: INDEPENDENCE	159
Karmic lesson 17: COURAGE	165
Karmic lesson 18: LOYALTY	173
Karmic lesson 19: DECISIVENESS	181
Karmic lesson 20: CREATIVITY	187
Karmic lesson 21: SOLITUDE	195
Karmic lesson 22: TEMPTATION	205
Karmic lesson 23: RESPECT	213
Epilogue	221

BRIGITTE CALLOWAY

ACKNOWLEDGMENTS

Thank you from the bottom of my heart to everybody who read my first book *"You have lived many times"*. Your encouragement was the trigger to write more.

This book would not have been possible without my clients' input; therefore I would like to thank to all my clients who trusted me in regressing them to past lives. It was an honor to witness your memories.

My gratitude goes to those whose cases are presented in this book. Unfortunately there are many others who I was not able to include. However, the future will prove that I haven't forgotten you.

I would like to thank my friend and proof reader Charlotte Giblin, who took the time to make my manuscript readable. Also to my husband who put up with how little spare time I had whilst writing this manuscript. Your constant encouragement means the world to me.

PROLOGUE

We are here to learn from each other

Nobody knows what happens behind closed doors other than the people who lock them. We all have secrets still left in the closet; some of which we have even forgot about. There may have been delightful - but forbidden - experiences or very powerful ones that affected us negatively. We put them in storage and hope that these things will never come out in the open. All of these experiences are related to people we came across at some stages in our lives. By hiding or even denying these memories, we protect ourselves from judgment and rejection.

    I was just two years old when my father gave me up for fostering. He was neither poor, nor cruel. Perhaps he thought that I was a constant reminder of his relationship with my mother, who left us when I was just a baby. I was therefore placed in the care of his sister and her husband. I can count on the fingers of one hand how many times I saw my father in my first twenty years of my life.

    The aunty who raised me became more than a mother to me, so soon after I arrived, I started calling her "mom". Everything I am now is because of her! I soon learnt that my new mom had her own secrets, which I inherited as a little girl and adopted as my own once I was part of her family. Unlike my father, my foster mother's family was very poor and it was hard for her and her husband to put food on the table for their children and me, the new child. And yet, nobody else knew this. Our neighbors perceived us as the wealthiest people in the suburb and most of our acquaintances envied us. Our poverty was something we never talked about and, once in our own home, we closed the doors behind us.

It was really easy to hide our social status because my mom taught us children - and demanded from us - high standards; she was an amazing dressmaker and she used to make us the most expensive looking garments. I was the only girl wearing a so-called "Chanel" suit or a copy of a Versace dress and that created envy amongst my peer group. My mom reproduced patterns perfectly and put her creative fingerprint on everything I wore. I remember that Sunday lunches consisted of so little food, but we celebrated them dressed up as queens and kings. We got out the finest china my foster parents could afford and laid the table with a beautiful white embroidered tablecloth. That taught me from a very early age to take enormous pride in my appearance… also to let people see only as much as I am willing to show them. As I have said, nobody knows what happens behind closed doors!

In our lives, we let our guard down with some people but not with others. We have an intuition that guides us to keep some people behind locked doors and to open them wide for others. This doesn't necessarily mean that some people are good for us whilst others are not. It just highlights the fact that our intuition tells us when and in front of whom we can let our hair down. We search for acceptance, tolerance and love more than anything else, and if this means we don't always show our true selves, so be it!

People influence us and we impact people. There may be love or hate involved, but in essence our existence leaves behind legacies that change the behavior of other humans. We are all here for the same reasons: to learn from some and teach others. We are all so similar, and yet, so different. We are all individuals seeking happiness. For some, being happy means accumulating material things; for others, building up an amazing career gives that feeling of being on top of the world. I am not sure what happiness means for you, but for me, being able to establish an intimate connection with fellow humans brings the peace I require to go further. For me, love is contagious and the source of everything good which can trigger higher experiences and ultimately create personal success.

Looking back at my life, I sometimes wonder why I met some people, who for a moment in time may have played a role in my life whilst also hurting me. What I understand now is that because of those people too, I evolved. My soul and their souls interacted for a fraction of time and, when our mission together was accomplished, we went separate ways. Therefore, as harsh as our connection may have seemed, it was still for my benefit, and hopefully for their benefit too.

Eager to find out more about human interactions, I based this book on relationships that started in past lives. Is it possible that we met some of our loved ones thousands of years ago, in a totally different existence? It is up to you to decide, but for me this is a certain fact.

This book focuses on the concept that we have lived many times together with people we know in the present, in a continuous cycle of accomplishing karmic lessons. In putting together this book, I picked some of the karmic assignments I felt were essential to understanding the process of rebirth.

All the cases presented have been recorded under hypnosis in my hypnotherapy practice. For privacy reasons, some of the names have been changed. In the hypnotic dialogue with my clients, I refer to myself as using the initials of my name, BC.

.

HOW WE REMEMBER PAST LIVES

"I never came upon any of my discoveries through the process of rational thinking"
Albert Einstein

My life changed the day my first book *"You have lived many times"* got published. The book created a fuss in the town where I lived and many people developed an interest in past lives, being prepared to explore their own healing journeys through past existences rather than continuing to use conventional approaches. Suddenly, client after client wanted to be regressed with the aim of getting closure on long lasting emotional and physical aches and pains. On top of my busy traditional hypnotherapy practice, I soon had to accommodate a large number of past life regression hypnosis requests. I was absolutely sure that healing through regression would have similar results to classical hypnotherapy for some clients.

Since *"You have lived many times"*, my working hours got longer, filled in not only with treating clients; but also with listening to the recordings made during trance and typing the hypnotic dialogues out on my laptop. Just when I started feeling more comfortable with my new hectic work schedule, people who read my first book contacted me asking for more. I got emails and messages practically demanding another book and the enthusiasm was contagious. I must confess I procrastinated for a few weeks, until one Saturday night I got a message from Stephen, one of my dear clients who worked offshore. I remembered that he bought a copy of *"You have lived many times"* and took it offshore, where he intended to read it and pass it on to his workmates, some of whom were already my clients. The message said *"your book is a best seller offshore.... it changes lives"*. Immediately after reading his message, I started working on this book.

You may wonder if past lives - the main concepts behind my whole approach - are real. Is it possible that we have lived many other times, even though we are unable to instantly and naturally recall memories from those lives? I believe that it is. As a hypnotherapist, I work with the human mind and I know that there is nothing as miraculous as the way the mind functions. Our brains act in a very similar way to our personalities or egos. Our minds bring forward what is relevant for our existence now in a similar manner to our spirits, filtering and using information and feelings according to specific situations. They keep a guard up in case of eventual danger, in the same way that we do when we sense the possibility of imminent harm, and let the guard down completely when everything seems fine.

Our brains store long term memories believed to be lost, which may seem irrelevant for our current existence, and permit others to come out, which are significant for who we are and what we are doing now. Our brains may recall a multitude of types of people who all seem familiar – be they black or white, poor or wealthy, healthy or handicapped, man or woman – because they are from our past lives and part of the same soul structure. The soul is unique and eternal, whilst each existence materializes in a different physical form. *"It is still Mary wearing different hats"*, as an old saying goes in my own culture.

The process of recalling memories is very similar to the process of thinking, if not the same. Imagine the state of continuous confusion your brain would experience if you could simultaneously remember all the memories from every life you have ever lived. In order to function with so-called *"peace of mind"*, the brain needs to keep to one side anything which is not essential, including any past life memories which might not correlate to the present moment. Because of this, when recalling past lives, a method of 'direct retrieval' cannot be used: memory association between past and present lives is complex and can be overwhelming. Just imagine how confused you would be if I asked you what you did on second September ten years ago. There is no way you could remember anything about that day, until I told you that second September was my birthday and you were one of my guests at a party I hosted in Fiji; these details may help you instantly remembering some details. If I went even further and started describing the other guests, the venue, the theme of the party, you would remember even more detailed aspects. What you may recall about that day might be totally different from what I remember, because we have individual perspectives on the same experience. However, for you to recall a vivid memory from that day in September, all I needed to do was to create associations for that day, which in turn enabled you to remember details with ease.

When it comes to past lives, the process of memory recall can sound more complex. For example, if I was to say that one of your past lives was in Egypt, your brain wouldn't be able to spontaneously correlate a memory from that specific life in Egypt if you hadn't travelled there in the present life, or done some research about the area. In a similar manner to the way a computer scans files, your brain would start scanning memories, but would not retrieve a past life memory from Egypt if it couldn't be associated with something you know from your present life. In the second instance, your brain would scan again searching for recognizable faces, and again, none of the people from the hypothetical past life in Egypt would mean anything whatsoever in the present. Therefore the 'face recognition phase' would also return with no results. It may seem like a complicated process, but it is not. It's a similar scenario to one in which you might try to find my grandmother's address without knowing her name or any relevant details about her or me. Imagine turning on your computer and entering in a search for *"Brigitto's grandmother's address"*. I can assure you that the search would come up with zero results because you were unable to supply the search engine with any of the main details needed for retrieving this specific information: recognition and association. You couldn't pinpoint a significant detail about my grandmother or me, other than my first name, and you were not able to associate and recall a fact about either of us. On top of that, there was no pre-existing memory of an event involving us, or a fact about us.

Distractions also prevent our brains from automatically retrieving past life memories, as they can affect the accuracy. Humans have 'distributive attention' which means that we divide our awareness according to main internal, external or environmental factors. During any experience, our attention is often divided between multiple points of focus: we're not just concentrating on the experience itself. This may affect or dissipate a memory we then try to recall at another moment in time. Just imagine the distractions caused by external factors that played a role in a specific experience in a past life, such as unknown people in that existence and historical habits or customs, and the distraction caused by any current external factors, in the moment you want to remember aspects from that long lost existence.

But perhaps the main reason you are not able to naturally remember anything whatsoever from a past life is down to your own brain activity. At the time you try to retrieve or recall a memory of an experienced fact, a place or people related to one of your past lives, your brain activity functions in beta brain waves. This is the state in which you are aware and able to maintain day-to-day activities. It is also the state people are spending the most time in. A long term memory that cannot be associated and wasn't used - or retrieved at least a few times - would not be able to be remembered instantly when your brain is working in beta waves. In the same way, your brain would not be capable of retrieving a memory while you are in a day dreaming state, which is a normal phase of relaxing and letting your mind go wild, as well as when you sleep, as this is a phase of unconsciousness when your brain emits gamma brainwaves. The only way of remembering such long term memories as those related to past lives, may be possible when your brain is functioning in theta waves, which is the main state of trance induced in hypnosis or very deep meditation.

I believe that there is no difference between remembering a long term memory in the present life and one that relates to a past life as long as your subconscious brain - the area where all long term memories are stored - can identify it by associating it with an already stored and perhaps recalled experience or functions in theta waves. It is one or the other really! Again, we remember naturally all kindred memories that have been used and utilized several times. Therefore, perhaps the only main distinction between recalling memories from a few years ago and hundreds of years ago is the state of brain activity in which the recollection takes place.

When I refer to recalling memories from past lives under hypnosis, I am alluding to retrospective memories that could be defined as *"recalling to remember"* or *"remembering to recall"*. The retrospective approach hinges on experiences from a distant past, which are continuing to have an impact now or will have in the future. Like any process of memory recall, a past life *"retrospective"* memory would most naturally appear as fragments, which you would try to piece together: small details would give clues to another part of the memory and trigger the next piece of the puzzle. On the other hand, a *"serial"* past life memory may be harder to recall, if not impossible, because the order of events would have to follow a more linear and chronological format, which would be much harder to match against any pattern in the present, or to find any 'association triggers'.

Imagine trying to find a file on your laptop. Your search would definitely take a long time if the file wasn't stored in an obvious place, with other files relating to the same topic; and it would take even longer if the file was very old – or in a hidden folder. If you haven't used that particular file recently or repetitively there would be no search history to assist you: accessing the file might be a difficult and time-consuming process, but ultimately it wouldn't be an impossible task.

To understand how a memory can be accessed, you first need to know how it is encoded and then stored. The hippocampus, an organ in the medial temporal lobe, is in charge of analyzing every input received from the sensory areas of the cortex, and ultimately deciding on the importance of each memory. Again, imagine the folders stored on the hard drive of your computer. Each file in each folder has been sorted and saved by you according to their content and association with other files, with the aim of fast and efficient access when required.

The process of encoding memories is based mainly on how they can be correlated and triggered by the four primary senses: visual, acoustic or audio, semantic or sensory and tactile. There is a common belief that long term memories are mostly based on the sensory encoding, which means that in a past life regression, a subject would mainly recall memories based on the feelings they have generated. This is perhaps the reason why most of my clients refer to memories in their regressions that created strong emotions. However, they might also have interpreted the memories through their own main representational systems in the present, which would then be subject to the most developed of their primary senses.

Once a memory is encoded, it has to be consolidated, stored, utilized and used in order to be accessed as a long term memory. In some cases, recalling the same memory more than once can create totally different feelings or emotions, which can be associated with other memories that generated the same sentiment. Again, picture the folders on the hard drive of your computer. You can change the location of a file anytime you want, once you add things to that file which alter its overall contents and change its context, or it develops similarities to files stored elsewhere.

All the experiences we can recall as memories are personal and are part of our individual consciousness, which may be referred to as *"tabula rasa"* if we believe that all our experiences stem from our perception and perspective. This concept of the mind's *"clean state"* was used by the ancient Greek Stoicism to explain and endorse the notion that our minds start with a blank page, before adding information impressed on us by external factors.

The psychoanalyst Carl Jung looked at the larger scale by developing the term of *"collective unconsciousness"*. Jung believed that humankind has a shared unconsciousness, based on archaic archetypes that are universal. Therefore, the personal unconsciousness would include memories that may have been forgotten or repressed, even if they have at some stage been part of our own individual awareness or consciousness; whilst the collective unconsciousness mainly refers to inherited presuppositions and symbols. This may emphasize the fact that we all have something in common even if we have different abilities and perceptions. For Jung, our existence relies on ego, which is the conscious part of our brains, and on personal and collective unconsciousness. All the symbols we inherited may therefore be grounded at our collective unconsciousness level. Jung's theory on the collective unconsciousness was acclaimed and criticized at the same time. It is up to you whether you believe in it or totally disagree with it. You won't be the first one to argue over it. Sigmund Freud contested Jung's view on the unconscious human mind. He believed that this is a space for traumatic memories and sex drive rather than a pre-existing and collective database of symbols. The controversy between the two goes far deeper anyway: their views differentiated on other subjects such as religion, dreams, and sexuality. For me, there is no right or wrong with regards to any of them, and what I take from both perspectives is the fact that our unconsciousness may have collective patterns based on belonging beliefs.

  You may ask yourself why we forget memories. I would suggest that 'forgetting' is a natural process, and also a temporary one. We don't forget experiences forever unless we suffer amnesia. Memories cannot be voluntarily deleted, as much as we would like to get rid of some really traumatic ones. Once stored as long-term memories, they can fade, but not disappear. They may seem forgotten only because they haven't been used or utilized enough.

  There is also another aspect to consider regarding the process of 'forgetting': the hippocampus, the main center in charge of sorting memories and learning, is the first part of our brains to deteriorate with age. This is perhaps the reason why children tend to connect and access memories from past lives more easily. There are so many cases of children who remember naturally and instantly previous existences. These children have been the subjects of research with no certain conclusion about why and how they remember past lives in the absence of trance. It is said that up to the age of six, we can all naturally remember facts from our previous lifetimes, but I am not sure I can prove this. What I do know however is that we were born with the ability to remember everything and, when we forget, we can 'learn how to remember'. Learning is just a way of remembering.

You may now agree that past life memories can be accessed, but still wonder whether or not you have lived more than once you might even be skeptical, or disagree entirely with this concept. This is something we may agree to disagree on! For me, past lives have been proven by my many clients who recalled detailed memories from existences other than the one they currently abide. They weren't dreams, fake memories or hallucinations. They were historically correct details that meant the world to their own souls. They recognized themselves and the energy of people they know in their current lives. The places and names sounded to them familiar and the events real.

I don't belong to any religious movements and I don't worship anything other than life itself. I don't base my life on any devotional beliefs or customs and I don't consider that the history of souls is confined to any particular belief system. I believe that the soul is immortal and that it reincarnates repetitively with the aim of evolving. I also believe that with every incarnation, souls get closer to excellence and have a higher chance of reaching perfection. Again, my evidence and understanding is based on numerous past life regression cases recorded in my practice.

If you believe that this life is the only one you have ever lived, I would challenge you to prove this belief! I would also suggest that you try having the experience of a past life regression, which would enable you to then draw a more considered conclusion. Deep down, I think we all feel that there must be more than just this one life!

SOUL GROUPS

"Great acts are made up of small deeds"
Lao Tzu

Many of my clients recalled with surprise and even stupefaction past life memories about people who are present in their current life. They didn't recognize their faces, bodies or personalities; but they knew their energies. For them, the interdependence with some people in the present was evident in a past existence as well. My clients recognized themselves in totally different bodies and this didn't make them feel uncomfortable at all. Strong and handsome men in my practice saw themselves in fragile women's bodies; elderly ladies remembered themselves in fit, muscular, manly bodies; clients with a light complexion recalled their dark skins and they all felt at ease with their appearances. You may wonder how these people were certain that, in a deep hypnotic trance, they had seen themselves and not somebody else; was this just a hallucination or a real memory? Well, I believe they acknowledged the presence of their energetic fields rather than their physical appearance.

We produce, use, absorb and emit energy. Our bodies are surrounded by energetic layers, which form our subtle body, called aura. It is at the aura level that we sense other people's energies, forming an instant sense of like or dislike before any sort of direct interaction. This first impression about a person can certainly change in time, but usually the initial impact is strong.

I am sure that you have heard about *"love at first sight"* and wondered what initiates the instant feeling of falling in love with someone you know nothing about. Is it a particular physical aspect one can suddenly and unexpectedly fall in love with or is the attraction at a much deeper level? I believe that our auras give out details about our mental and emotional status prior to proper interaction. You may call this intuition or gut feeling; I however believe that it is the interaction of our energetic fields.

Without going into too much depth, I want to mention that it is believed that our subtle body contains seven layers of energy, each varying in size and depth and each connected to one of our seven main energy organs situated inside our bodies, called chakras. Each aura level has its own vibration. The seven layers are: the Etheric body, the Emotional body, the Mental body, the Astral body, the Etheric Template, the Celestial body and the Ketheric Template. Each layer transmits details about our mental, emotional and physical self-awareness. It is said that our interaction, interdependence and coexistence with others starts with the vibrations sensed at the Astral energetic level, because this layer acts like an overpass between the physical and spiritual aspects of any being.

As our auras extend to two or even three meters away from the physical body, we can sense details of another person when we enter their energetic field. So, from six meters away, two people can feel each other's emotional energies and can make an instant judgment about one another. It is simply another form of communication between people, like language, body language and even silence.

Anytime I talk about the energetic layers that surround our bodies, one of my friends comes to my mind. We were best friends in high school, both very young and fearless. One Saturday evening we attended a party, hosted by one of our schoolmates. We arrived at the same time, and as we entered the house we couldn't see the faces of the other youngsters very clearly. We recognized a few people but there were also a lot of unfamiliar faces. A few minutes later, my buddy was stood staring at one of the corners of the room, where a girl was talking to some friends of ours. I couldn't see her face in the semi-darkness and neither could he. Suddenly, my best friend said *"I will marry that girl"* and you know what? He started dating her, and right after graduation, he married her. They are still together and very happy. At their wedding, I asked him what he saw in his bride-to-be and how was he instantly sure that she was 'the one'? I remember his answer very clearly: *"I just knew, the second I laid eyes on her"*. Were they communicating to each other through their auras or was it just a stubborn love? I don't have the answer, but I do know that anything is possible.

The process of recognizing people involved in our past lives could well be based on the feel of their energetic fields. Despite having a different outward appearance, their energies may have seemed very similar to their present incarnations. My clients recalled memories in which their past-life grandfathers have become their present-life mothers, or their past-life husbands have become their present-life children, and this introduces the idea of soul groups.

The whole concept of 'soul groups' is based on the idea of continuous reincarnations with the same group of people; each member of the group plays a different role in each lifetime, and has specific connections depending on the karmic lessons each soul has decided to accomplish. Therefore soul groups can be said to be *"perpetuum mobile"* connections. Some believe that there are main or primary soul groups that travel together in each life; others speak about secondary and even tertiary soul groups. They all agree however that the connections we establish with some souls are not random, but instead they are purposefully arranged in order to achieve a high level of development on both sides. I agree that in order for a relationship to evolve to the highest possible level, some souls may be part of each other's lives for many consecutive existences, whilst others may achieve their intended purpose in one existence only. I suppose that there is no 'one rule' with regards to interdependence and coexistence.

Whether you believe in reincarnation or you haven't made up your mind about it just yet, you may wonder how much you can trust the concept of meeting your loved ones again in other existences. Well, to my knowledge this can only happen for the pure purpose of evolution. What I mean is that the soul's motivation and purpose is to grow, develop and advance. Don't we desire progress as humans too? We come into the world as babies with survival instincts, and then we learn during our existence about boundaries, punishment, independence, relationships, achievement and autonomy. Based on our beliefs and habits that we have inherited from the cultures we belong to, we grasp at and try to attain knowledge about how to grow independently as well as how to co-exist with others; how to achieve physically, emotionally, intellectually and materially according to our circumstances and situations. As strong and determined as we may be, we cannot develop to our true potential without interacting with other humans. We need their knowledge and experience as much as we need their support, love, and empathy - and sometimes even their rejection. We grow as others do too. We are influenced by the evolution of others, as we impact others also.

The soul's evolution follows the same patterns as we - spirits - do. Souls need to interact with other souls in order to mature in the same manner as us - spiritual beings - require interconnection. This can be accomplished in each life through what we describe as good or bad experiences. Just because somebody affects your present life negatively it doesn't mean that they have created obstructive or harmful ripples throughout the history of your soul. Your immortal soul may have achieved more by going through a disaster: at the soul's level this may have been an immense step forward. Through favorable and adverse situations, the soul learns and evolves with each lesson fulfilled. You have lived many lives because your soul has needed to grab knowledge from others and pass on skills to fellow souls.

One approach to understanding reincarnation is to recognize how similar it is to the way we interpret commercial advertisements seen on screen. As we all know, products are presented to us with a web of our own expectations wrapped around them. I love watching commercials because, in order to produce sales, in just a few seconds, a clip has to tell a story about a dream product and how to use it, as well as responding to all the potential questions we may have. Smart commercials are built around one true fact, covered in layers of fiction. It fascinates me how a few words said in the right manner can grasp our attention and keep us, watchers, excited about the product. A commercial could be an analogy for what we understand about souls and their evolutions. Starting with what we all know about evolving as a desirable and achievable state for humankind, we design a whole network of suppositions, expectations and assumptions, imagining that they all carry the same meaning for our eternal souls as for our physical existence.

What seems contradictory is the idea that a negative experience in one of our existences could lift a soul higher on the soul's hauraki. This is based on the lessons a soul is supposed to learn through - and in - each lifetime. None of these 'assessments' can be achieved in the absence of interactions with other souls: to be able to solve equations and algorithms, one has to first learn the numbers, and then how these can be added, multiplied and divided. To be a mathematician, one first learns the basics and then advances by learning as many details as possible related to numeracy. In the same way, souls have to learn about each situation and experience at the physical, emotional and spiritual levels.

Evolution itself is nothing other than applied encyclopedic facts. Imagine getting an encyclopedia when you first incarnated and passing exams for each life you have ever lived. It takes time and patience to read the encyclopedia and apply all the knowledge. All of us were given the same book, but each of us understands it in a different way and expresses the content in an individual and unique manner. Sometimes we read it together; other times alone. However, we all do master it in our own time and apply the knowledge we gained according to our own abilities, skills and specific circumstances.

Some believe that we die when we finish learning our primary lesson, because our mission has been accomplished. I am not sure I agree with this, and I could debate the topic for hours. What I believe is that death is neither random, nor coincidental as life itself is not. I also agree that 'crossing over' may come at a certain point, agreed to by our souls just before being incarnated or reincarnated. Our souls may have signed the contract of life and death alone, in the presence of other souls or even co-signed with other souls.

In my opinion, there is another reason why some souls reincarnate in the same groups. I believe that, in each existence, other souls give our incarnated spirits a feeling of familiarity. Even if we forget about our common experiences in other lives, we recognize their familiarity. I believe that our relationships with others are based on that. We feel connected because we unconsciously know that our life paths have crossed at some stage in another existence perhaps, or that we belong to something bigger, even if we cannot put our finger on what that may be. We adopt shared existences for a while if we sense common interests. Just remember how you chose your friends in the early stages of your childhood. In kindergarten for instance, your friends were children who liked the same toys and games. Without having any knowledge about the other children in general, you picked those you felt familiar with and who shared the same focus. Then later in school, you chose friends who had common interests in what was important for you, either sports or music for instance. They may have had a totally different upbringing or belonged to other races or cultures, but the child in you recognized the desire to be in their environment because you felt familiarity through shared likes and dislikes. Then, when you picked your life partner, I don't believe that it was only your heart that dictated the choice of one person over another. We unconsciously choose people who make us feel comfortable in our own skins.

The topic of déjà vu always pops up when we refer to familiarity. Some research into the topic defines the two as having the same reference and meaning. In my opinion, the concept of déjà vu is the awareness of our consciousness in regards to distinguishing pattern similarities. Our systems of values, beliefs and habitual similitude recollect and recognize homogeneous structures that may have coexisted in other lives. *"I have the feeling that I know you from somewhere"* may not always mean that we have met before in our current existence; it may symbolize that our energies have come across one another way before that, perhaps in a past life. The feeling may be deep and may create a wave of familiar energy that I like to define as déjà vu. The emotion is even stronger if both souls convey it in a romantic manner. This is where soul mates or twin souls may have a purpose, but these are controversial subjects too. Despite what I read about soul mates and twin souls, my definition is based on my own experiences with past life regressions. Again, all of these occurrences are filtered though my clients' memories from past lives.

I believe that we have several soul mates, all of whom play diverse roles in different lifetimes; with a slim chance, if any, of a purely romantically connotation. A soul mate can be any person we deeply relate to, if we both evolve from our coexistence or interdependence. Our evolution doesn't necessarily have to be at a spiritual level though. One can define a friend, relative, partner, teacher and even a pet as a soul mate and to be perfectly honest all these hypostases can coexist. However, a twin soul guides two souls to a spiritual achievement. The emotional relationship of the two can be shaky, whilst the growth in awareness remarkable. I have met many people who assumed that their 'on and off' relationship with a lover might have defined them as twin souls. I believe that twin souls serve each other's spiritual enlightenment – two people with an unstable relationship and lack of long-term emotional common ground doesn't necessarily equal twin souls.

It is said that twin souls are derived from a division of the same soul. The two halves therefore mirror each other, making the connection difficult. In my opinion, in most cases, a relationship between twin souls is more of a curse than a blessing.

You may find the whole concept of soul groups - involving soul mates, twin souls and kindred souls - a little bit confusing, or you may totally disagree with it. You may also think that déjà vu is a subject mostly related to fantasy. Again, there is no right or wrong in a territory that is not fully understood or explored yet. I assume that we would both agree, however, that evolution is the main aim of humankind. I would go even further and argue that the same concept defines the desire and goal of each soul. As I have said previously, this can be achieved by pursuing life lessons in each existence. At the end of the day, learning never finishes. There is always something more to assimilate and master and there are always various perspectives to the whole learning process. All of these aspects are connected and ultimately form our own consciousness.

There are many lessons a soul has to accomplish in each life. Some people call them karmic lessons, others destiny paths. No matter how you refer to them, each of these assignments is part of evolution and enlightenment. Your soul therefore has to master how to function independently as well as coexisting with others; how to understand itself and others; how to connect in small and large groups; how to love itself and others. Each of these aspects are, in my opinion, based on the concepts of love, tolerance, compassion and empathy; the ultimate goal being raising self-awareness and contributing positively to the collective consciousness. In essence, all the assignments our souls have to pass could be resumed to understanding that we are all part of the universe that is one with us.

Many of my clients often ask *"what is the highest level a soul can evolve to?"* In other words, when is the soul good enough for itself and universality and no longer needs to reincarnate to learn more. To be honest, I cannot answer this question because I believe that there is always another lesson added to our development with the evolution of the planet itself. However, I don't deny the fact that some souls may have reached perfection and don't need to reincarnate again. I cannot argue whether these high souls have been avid learners and evolved faster, or whether they have been chosen as master souls at their own formation. For me, the possibilities are endless and never coincidental.

KARMA AND KARMIC LESSONS

"For every action, there is an equal opposite reaction"
Isaac Newton

Karma is one of the most controversial subjects, and not just for those who believe in reincarnation. We tend to use the term in order to emphasize that there is a bigger picture we all are a part of, and a higher force that would reward or punish our actions. In fact, we apply it in a manner that serves us to approve or disapprove with our actions or the actions of others. For most people, karma is an assurance that the Universe is in charge and will respond to our actions. Therefore, we remember about karma when it assists us, by criticizing somebody else's behavior and excusing ours.

Karma is not the Damocles sword, suspended over our heads by a single hair; therefore not an act of punishment. Karma is in fact a law of cause and effect, stipulating that every action initiates at least one consequence. I usually explain karma to my clients by relating it to weight loss. If they overeat and are not keeping themselves active, one of the results could be gaining weight, or in other words, we initiate what happens to us. As simple as that!

We cannot accept the validity of karma if we deny Samsara, rebirth or reincarnation, and the role played by our own free will in the cycle of lives. These three concepts work together in symbiosis. But before I go into depth, I need to advise you, my readers, that I am not a follower of any of the existent religions or divinization beliefs. I am not a New Age adept either and I don't adhere to any worshiping doctrine. My personal beliefs are based on my studies and my work regarding past life regressions. Therefore, they may not be universal. It is up to you to agree or disagree with my individual perspective.

Karma is based on the concept of reincarnation, according to which our souls may be eternal and come back to more than one existence in order to reach perfection. Many religions, like Hinduism, Buddhism, Jainism and Sikhism, established their beliefs on reincarnation. Their views may differ on the material perpetuated or carried from life to life, but they all agree that there is more than this life we are living at the present time.

The etymology of reincarnation doesn't find its roots in Sanskrit as one would expect; it actually comes from the Latin *"reincarnationem"*, which means *"entering again"*, referring to the soul entering flesh or body furthermore. Even the origin of this concept is far from belonging to ancient Indian religious dogma, because the same idea of reincarnation is present in the pre-Socratic philosophy. However the most cited reference of the notion of reincarnation is in the Upanishads.

Over the years, I have noticed that people very often confuse the Upanishads with the Vedas. For a little clarity, I would say that the Vedas are ancient Sanskrit religious texts, believed to be transmitted from the god Brahman, and correlated to the main scriptures that are followed in Hinduism. The Vedas, referring to the word *"knowledge"* in Sanskrit, originated around 1500BC and consist of four main areas of knowledge required for spiritual development: Rig-Veda, based on hymns used for recitation; Sama-Veda, built on specific teachings of sounds or melodies for chanting; Yajur-Veda, incorporating details on specific rituals; and Atharva-Veda, based on everyday procedures or routines. Some of these parts of the Vedas comprise of hymns, other of mantras or ritual formulas.

On the other hand, the Upanishads are a collection of hymns, considered to be of a philosophical nature because of their approach to the unity of Atman, the soul, and Brahman, the universal source. The Upanishads are believed to be created by *"rishis"*, who, according to Hinduism, were *"Jogis"* or *"sages"* and who received the supreme knowledge in meditation. It is in the Upanishads that Samsara and the concept of 'good deed being repaid' was mentioned first.

If Hinduism agrees with reincarnation in a very particular way, death being followed by a heavenly life and a second death, for Buddhism the soul is not endless and karmic lessons are not passed from one life to another. Therefore with each reincarnation only the knowledge is carried on, while with every life a new materialized spirit is created. This cycle of life and death for Buddhism finishes once Nirvana, or enlightenment, is reached; this being the supreme escape from karma. For Jainism, rebirth has one ultimate aim: liberation. The same liberation is sought in Sikhism, based on the concept of karma accumulated in a life that determines the next reincarnation.

If the approach to the cycle of numerous incarnations is pretty similar - whilst the interpretation of it may differ - the concept is straightforward: after death, a soul reincarnates with the aim of reaching that supreme state in which it can escape the cycle. For some religions, rebirth is based on karma accumulated in a previous life or even arbitrarily; for me though, it is the soul that decides on the necessity of the next incarnation based on how it can achieve a specific assignment. In my opinion, there are multitudes of karmic lessons, all based on different scenarios, circumstances and our free will in each life.

The concept of free will doesn't belong only to religious movements that embrace reincarnation and karma; it is also present in Christianity. Christians believe that people have the freedom to sin or not, choose heaven or hell, and therefore to believe in God. For Judaism, the notion of free will is strongly related to divine creation; humankind being constructed to believe in and rejoice with God itself. Even Kabala admits the possibility of free will, and afterlife is based on the choices made in a lifetime. These choices themselves determine our present karma according to Hinduism.

The freedom to choose between good and bad is a paradox for one who believes that everything is predestined. However, free will and predestination may coexist simultaneously. I believe that what is meant to be will be, only if one chooses the right path that makes this possible. To be perfectly honest, a life predestined in every aspect may be boring, for me at least. In my opinion, choosing one lesson over another was made by our own souls before reincarnation, and the way we complete it is based on our free will after incarnation. In other words, we may be meant to meet our twin soul for instance, but it is up to us to search for it or not.

We like to believe that if we do a good act we will receive one in response; also that a wealthy and healthy life is the effect of a previous life in which we built up predominantly good karma, whist an unfortunate life is caused by bad karma accumulated in a past life. I hope that I am not disappointing you when I say that things don't work exactly like that. Just because somebody is born with a severe handicap it doesn't mean that in a previous life that person may have done every evil thing possible, which added up to balance their bad karma against the good. I am not even sure that we can refer to karma as good and bad. Karma is in a state of permanent change; it is neither good, nor bad; it is only a sum of effects to our actions during each life we have ever lived.

When we mention karma, we have to acknowledge that karma works on three levels: one that we construct in the present life, another one that is accumulated in every life we have lived so far - including the present one - and a component of it that is already in action, so it cannot be stopped. So things are never straightforward with regards to positive and negative, but what is really clear is that the way our ego expresses itself now, affects our path in the future. The famous psychoanalyst Carl Jung argued that *"I do not know whether karma creates the ego or the ego creates karma"*. At the end of the day the source of unhappiness may be an implemented belief rather than the effect of our actions.

Karmic lesson 1

LOVE

"To love and let go"

I met Julie a while ago and I wasn't surprised at all when she booked a past life regression session. I heard from some mutual friends that she had been through a hard time lately, but didn't want to ask them for details. Julie's appointment was my last before the Christmas holidays and I remember that hot and sunny day. Christmas falls in full summer here, in New Zealand. I also remember how excited I was about having two weeks off right after Julie's appointment. As I prepared the room for the session, I tried recalling her face. I knew for sure that she was young, but as I have only met her once a long time ago, no details came back to me.

Julie arrived right on time and I noticed that she was young indeed, maybe in her early thirties, and very well presented. I knew that she worked in the natural medical field and that she was very successful. As she started talking, I realized how much I liked her: she was smart, very polite and had a soft way of being. Her voice was as delicate as her body was.

I let her talk for a while before asking what the reason was behind wanting to go through a regression. Tears started falling down her beautiful face and her body seemed smaller whilst she told me about her brother who passed away traumatically just a few months ago. She said that she missed him and felt so hopeless without him. Whilst Julie shared memories about her brother, I realized that she believed it was unusual for him not to communicate in any manner with her, even after passing over. Julie believed in life after life and couldn't understand why the relationship with her brother stopped after his death. She was wondering whether their connection started in a past life and their mission together finished in the present life.

As Julie talked about her belief in reincarnation and about the special bond with her brother, I forgot that in less than two hours, my two week holiday would start. I was mesmerized by her beautiful personality and wanted to help her as much as I was able to. I started inducing hypnosis and the whole process was *"a la carte"*. As Julie's body relaxed, she looked even more pleasant; she was in great shape and very fit. When I began asking questions, I hoped that Julie would revisit a lifetime that would have been relevant enough for her to make peace in her heart.

BC: *"What do you see, hear or feel?"*

Julie: *"I am a monk. I am wearing sandals and a brown robe. I am walking on a road."*

BC: *"Can you remember your name?"*

Julie: *"My name is Brian."*

BC: *"So you are waking on a road. Do you know where you are going?"*

Julie: *"It is quiet.... only me walking.... and a woman. I think that I am going to where I belong.... where the monks live."*

BC: *"Tell me about that woman."*

Julie: *"She is beautiful. She is in her thirties. She has green eyes and blonde hair. She wears a long dress. I remember that she was someone I loved."*

BC: *"Is she somebody you know in the present?"*

Julie kept quiet for a while, and then she started smiling. Her face lit up when she answered.

Julie: *"Yes. She is my brother."*

I knew that she referred to her lost brother and I was happy that she decided to revisit a lifetime in which he was present. That would perhaps bring her hope that they could be together again in the future.

BC: *"Do you remember why you became a monk?"*

Julie: *"Because of that woman. She didn't hurt me. She was taken away from me. Her family married her to an older, very wealthy man. I loved her! Her name starts with an N.... maybe Naurelle."*

BC: *"Tell me about the monastery."*

Julie: *"There are at least twenty monks living there. I don't feel connected to any of them. For sure there is no connection between us..."*

BC: *"Can you remember the year?"*

Julie: *"The year is 1541.... I am somewhere in Denmark."*

BC: *"Let's now go back in time, whilst I count down from three to one, to a moment when you were younger and in love with that woman."*

Whilst I was counting, I caught with the corner of my eye a black bird stopping in front of my window. The bird's wings stayed still for a moment, so I turned my head, looked at it and thought to myself that it would have flown in the room if the window was open. It was one of the hottest summers I have ever experienced in New Zealand and nature was blooming. The grass and flowers loved the sun and the humidity. Whilst still focusing on the bird that stopped in front of my window, I remembered that very soon my holiday would start and I felt instantly happy. As

Julie kept quiet, in an effort to remember details about her life in Denmark, my mind wandered to things I would love to do in the summer holiday: decorating the Christmas tree, cooking the most amazing meals for the festive day, walking my dog on the beach.... Then Julie began talking again with her soft, pleasant voice.

Julie: *"I am a servant, just a young boy.... aged... eighteen. She is at a similar age. I am a servant to her family. We love each other. We feel so carefree. Her sister found out about us. She is older. She feels so familiar, but I don't know exactly who she is."*

BC: *"No problem. Do you remember having any siblings?"*

Julie: *"I have a younger brother who works with me as a servant. He knows too about me and the girl I love."*

BC: *"Do you recognize him?"*

Julie: *"Yes, he is my father now."*

Julie's father passed away when she was a young girl. Suddenly, I remembered that she mentioned him and the close relationship they had. I was filled with joy that she remembered a past life with him.

BC: *"Tell me what happens."*

Julie: *"They married my lover to that older man. I was at her wedding... as a servant. Her dress was white and long. So beautiful! After the wedding, we kept seeing each other. Then something happened... we were found again. Her sister found out about us."*

BC: *"Think about her sister and try to remember if she is somebody you know in the present life."*

Julie: *"My niece... my brother's daughter."*

I couldn't stop thinking about how lucky Julie was revisiting a life with all the people she loved at the moment and, to be honest, this session was a success so far.

BC: *"What happened after you were found?"*

Julie: *"I was beaten badly. She remained in the marriage. Her family kept everything a secret. I thought that I had to become a monk. I knew I couldn't love again..."*

BC: *"I want you to go now to the very last moments of that life, just before dying and, when you are there, I want you to tell me how old you are."*

Julie: *"I am in my eighties. I am in the same monastery... very miserable... There are monks around, but I cannot connect with them. I am thinking about the woman I once loved. I never heard from her again. Somebody told me that she had two children, a girl and a boy."*

BC: *"Just focus on them. Do you recognize them?"*

Julie: *"The girl I don't know... the boy is my nephew now."*

BC: *"I want you to experience your soul leaving your body and, as you do that, maybe remember if there was any contract or promise you made in that lifetime and carried it into the present."*

Julie: *"Yes. Between me and her... to always love her."*

BC: *"I want you to break that promise and leave it behind. Now let your soul float higher and higher to the place where it is going to be healed. And whilst you do that, can you remember the lesson you learnt in that lifetime?"*

Julie: *"To love unconditionally and to let go... yes, to love and let go!"*

I knew that there was nothing else to be said, so I brought Julie back to complete awareness. She kept quiet for a while, and then tears of happiness started falling down her beautiful face. I wanted badly to know if she found her answers and if the regression helped her heal the pain of loosing her brother. Julie said that she now knew that her bond with her brother started very long time ago, in 1541 in Denmark. I was wondering how many other lives they might have had together.

Julie and I chatted for quite a while, so I tried answering all her questions about the journey of a soul in past lives. I however knew that she held the key to her soul's travel in time. Julie mostly doubted that she completely let go of the woman she loved hundreds of years ago and decided to fix in the present what she couldn't fix in the past. She said that it was the right time to focus on the beautiful moments she had with her brother rather than desperately holding his memory alive. Julie's past life regression made her realize that her brother was gone and, no matter how hard she tried, he wouldn't come back to this life. She felt relieved and I sensed that her life might change in an instant as she realized that any communication with him, other than in spirit, was not possible in this life. However, her brother's son and daughter are part of her life now. Their relationship started too in the lifetime when she was a young servant in love with a beautiful girl.

It is common to remember your loved ones in past lives; at least according to my clients' experiences in their regressions. Some of them have sensed their spouses, children or parents as part of other existences, whilst others have felt the presence of current friends or even neighbors in a life they forgot about. For Julie, her brother was a lover in another lifetime, whilst his current children were also part of the same existence. Her soul group incarnated together in more than one life and this gave her assurance that the same phenomenon may happen all over again.

I often remember Julie and wonder whether she had to repeat a karmic lesson in the present life. If in 1541, Julie's incarnation as a monk had to achieve unconditional love and learn to let go of it, nowadays it seemed as if she had to come back to gain more understanding of loving her brother and then let him go one more time when he crossed over.

I believe that there may be a possibility of repeating some karmic lessons even when they appear to be fully achieved initially. Perhaps revisiting karmic lessons may appear as passing exams at school or university. Sometimes a B mark is not good enough for one who strives for an A plus. Similarly, perhaps one soul can settle on a plan of action to relearn the same lesson all over again until it is achieved with excellence.

But what are these lessons our souls come to earth to achieve? Well, everything that uplifts our personal consciousness and contributes to the universal awareness could be an exam to pass. Many people refer to eleven main karmic lessons: independence, trust, balance, hard work, temptation, addictions, loyalty, family, empathy, prosperity, fear, spirituality and Impact on the world. Again based on my clients' regressions, I believe that there may be many more. I also believe that there are unlimited scenarios that may help us accomplish a lesson based on the way one is prone to learn.

In my opinion, love is behind all the possible karmic lessons, because we can conquer the world if we achieve unconditional love. There is nothing more assiduous than giving love to people who may not deserve it, and even harder to receive love from the ones who hurt us in the past. However, love may be the foundation of evolution itself and sometimes I wonder if love is actually the only lesson we have to learn, through unusual experiences in repetitive lives.

I have to admit that the term of *"unconditional love"* is trendy these days and comes across in everything that media manifests in. It is no wonder that 'love' is the top keyword searched on the Internet. Every religious or agnostic belief is based on love and every dogma starts with the principle of love. In my opinion, love and trust are the first emotions we experience when we are born. I am not sure whether it is love at first sight when we first see our mothers, but I agree that we start trusting them right after the first time we are breastfed. Perhaps mothers understand best what unconditional love is, but again I cannot generalize. Some do; others don't.

In my opinion, no human is able to deeply love unconditionally. We acknowledge feelings and circumstances on a personal basis and we respond individually to them. What is love for me may be different for you. I know for sure that we crave to be loved unconditionally, but we may not be able to reciprocate. We are in search of love our whole lives. We seek careers we think we love and we pursue relationships with people we are in love with. And perhaps because we base our existences on fondness, love may be the most common term we use in our own vocabulary. We *"would love"* to have a meal with friends, have a rest when we are tired, meet new people and spend time with old acquaintances. I sometimes wonder how love could transform into hate in an instant, because in the name of love we create masterpieces and yet we also start wars. And with love written all over their faces, some people uplift others; some kill them.

Therefore, lately I've been pondering how can we fall out of love, if passionate love was the initial feeling we had for someone because, let's be honest here, we cannot fall out of unconditional love. Perhaps what we call love sometimes is nothing else than just a temporary phase of lust. For me - not that I can affirm that I was ever able to love someone unconditionally other than my children - love comprises every positive feeling and human action: trust, tolerance, acceptance, encouragement, forgiveness, empathy and so many more. Therefore, it is the hardest to achieve.

Many believe that unconditional love starts with accepting and loving who they are, and they may be right, as long as self-love is not an actual form of narcissism or selfishness. For people to connect, gel and deepen their relationships, they may have to change and accommodate other people's needs. It's just the way love works. I strongly believe that we are able to give unconditional love once we understand that it is a virtue more than a feeling.

No matter whether we refer to love as *"agape"* in Christianity, *"karuna"* or *"kama"* in Buddhism, *"prema"* in Hinduism or *"athava"* in Judaism, love is the primordial feeling our souls are meant to experience on earth. In all these, love is a sacrament that allows unification with God, perceived as being a form of pure love itself. Therefore, the way to salvation is paved with unconditional love.

Karmic lesson 2

SUCCESS

"Just do it!"

I am extremely particular about my shoes and I meticulously pick out ones that are less likely to be worn by others, so I was surprised to see Moira owning a pair like mine. This was the first thing I noticed when she came in for her appointment.

I met Moira more than a year ago and instantly liked everything about her. She oozed confidence and energy and she knew who she was. Each of her gestures was a calculated result of self-trust and determination to be authentic. And she was exactly that; there was nothing fake about Moira!

I knew that she worked in high management and I had followed her success over the last year. Moira was terrific in her career and a very special woman outside of work! In her fifties, Moira was a beautiful woman. Perfectly styled blonde hair, great fashion taste, elegant, sophisticated - but casual when needed; she had it all! Her forte though was her atypical intelligence and exceptional communication skills.

She didn't tell me why she wanted to be regressed and I didn't push for details when she phoned to book the appointment. I suspected there was something that had been bothering her lately or perhaps a small detail was out of alignment in her very logical life. Therefore, this was the first question I asked when we sat down in my practice. Her answer was quite vague, so I decided to leave things the way they were and start the session.

Moira proved to me again that it was a piece of cake to induce trance with somebody who wanted to be hypnotized. Things get more complex with resistant clients, but Moira wasn't one of them. Her body relaxed quickly and, just a few minutes later, she began her journey in one of her past lives.

Moira: *"I see oak trees... tall oak trees. It's daytime."*

BC: *"Look down at your feet. How do they look; smaller, bigger, perhaps the same?"*

Moira: *"They are bigger and dirty because I am walking on a path. I am a man. I am going somewhere... I am going towards a house... a very old house, but happy house. I am going home. My family is there."*

BC: *"Tell me about your family."*

Moira: *"There are little children in the house. I have a happy family, but we have no money. I work on the land. I have rabbits that I killed. That's dinner..."*

BC: *"Do you remember your name?"*

Moira: *"Jack. My wife's name is Elena."*

BC: *"Is she somebody you know in the present?"*

Moira: *"Not her, but one of my boys is one of my boys now... the youngest one. His name is Jack Junior. He is six."*

BC: *"How old are you?"*

Moira: *"Hmm ... twenty-five... twenty-six years old."*

BC: *"As I count from three to one, I want you to go to a scene in that lifetime that is relevant to you."*

I expected to hear more about Jack's family when I started counting down. Moira proved once again that in a regression, even my expectations can be unrealistic suppositions. The memories that came back were from a totally different lifetime which she decided to revisit.

Moira: *"I am in a snowstorm. It's not... France?... it's a Slavic country. It's dark. It is cold, but I am not afraid. I am only ten. I have to find my house, but it's dark."*

BC. *"What do you remember about your family?"*

Moira: *"My mother's name is Steph. We have got more money in this family. My father sits in a chair next to the fire. He holds a pipe in his hand."*

BC: *"Do you recognize any of their energies?"*

Moira: *"My father is my grandfather now. He is funny. We are close allies against the mother. He gives me a wink."*

I decided on the spot to do things my way. I knew that there was more to know about Jack and his family and I wasn't prepared to let those memories slip away.

BC: *"I want you now to go back to the lifetime as Jack. Take your time and find your way back. Are you there yet?"*

I already knew that Moira would surprise me again. And she did.

Moira: *"Yes. I am only two years old. I am so small... I am in the hall of a castle with my parents. I don't know why we are there. Everybody is very quiet. I see flags. My parents work for the owners of this castle."*

BC: *"Do you have siblings?"*

Moira: *"Not with me."*

BC: *"Now find yourself in a scene as an older Jack."*

Moira: *"I am thirty years old. I am not in the same place. I am closer to the castle, but it's on the way to another town. When I look at my feet now, I have shoes on... with buckles. Hmm... I believe that the castle belongs to me now. I am rich. I am fulfilled, taller, stronger, accomplished. I made it. I have the money to help others. I can make people happy."*

BC: *"How did you make your money?"*

Moira: *"Making swords. Supplying swords. I traded everything... silk... spices... I made it!"*

BC: *"What year is it?"*

Moira: *"In the 1500s."*

BC: *"What's happened to your wife and children?"*

Moira: *"They are still here. My children are growing up. My family is so happy we don't have to struggle anymore."*

BC: *"What happened to the little Jack Junior?"*

Moira: *"He takes over the business. My daughter opened a shop. My wife is doing very well.... she is so happy. I made it!"*

BC: *"Happy life, I guess. Now I want you to remember the last moments in the lifetime as Jack; the very last moments before dying."*

Moira: *"I am in my late fifties. I can't be bothered... it's time to go. I am sick... I am coughing. My lungs are not good. My family is so sad. They are all here with me while I am dying."*

BC: *"As you look back at your lifetime do you have any regret?"*

Moira: *"I am wondering if one of my younger boys is going to be fine. He just mucks around. He doesn't do anything."*

BC: *"Do you recognize his energy?"*

Moira: *"Yes, he is my grandson now."*

Moira kept silent. I waited for a few minutes, hoping that she would share more memories from her lifetime as Jack, but there was nothing else she seemed to remember. I looked at my shiny clock on the wall and realized that there was enough time to regress her to another existence. I hoped that Moira would surprise me with exciting memories.

BC: *"Whenever you are ready, let your soul jump into another body and another lifetime. Let me know if this happens."*

Moira: *"I see a woman with a cap on her head... like an old bonnet. It's who I am... I wear a brown long skirt."*

BC: *"How old are you?"*

Moira: *"I feel old, but I am only forty-three years old. My name is Marie."*

BC: *"Do you know where you are?"*

MM: *"I am in the mountains... in France. Trees are not doing well... they are whitish- grey wood... not quite dead, but they are not doing very well. I am not doing very well either."*

BC: *"Tell me what you are doing in the mountains."*

Moira: *"Remedies for all sorts of ailments. People are traveling long distances to get my remedies. I can't be bothered seeing so many people. I am a moody and grumpy woman. I feel like saying 'leave me alone'..."*

BC: *"Move now to another scene in that lifetime, one that is important for you."*

Moira: *"I feel warmer. I am in a rocking chair. I have a stick in my hand. I am standing up now. I am going out to people. Oh wow! I am in Portugal now. I make wine... port. I own a winery."*

Moira seemed surprised of her good fortune. Then suddenly she started crying. Her whole body posture changed and her face seemed in sufferance. Her voice was very low when she talked again whilst tears fell down her face.

Moira: *"He's going to get run over by a horse. There is nothing I can do about it..."*

BC: *"Who is he?"*

Moira: *"My partner. He is my ex husband in the present. I recognize him. My daughter is there. She is helping him. He got run over. I am boiling water for him. He has broken some bones."*

I kept looking at Moira whilst she was sharing her memory about a partner in a past life. I knew she was suffering and I remembered why. Her husband died a few years ago and I wasn't sure if she had gotten over the tragedy. It must have been very hard for her remembering that he may have died with her in other existences too, so I decided to move her attention away from him.

BC: *"Don't worry. Maybe move to another scene. Tell me what else is happening?"*

Moira: *"There are people sneaking in where we make the port. This is not good news. I think they want to sabotage. I know the people who run the other winery. They are ruthless."*

BC: *"Do you know who they are in the present?"*

Moira: *"They are the people I worked for a few years ago."*

BC: *"Tell me about what you see."*

Moira: *"I have to get some help. I call my friends and my neighbors for help. They are threatening them to stay away. They have done enough! They stay away. They know we know..."*

BC: *"I want you to move now to the very last moment of this lifetime. Where are you now?"*

Moira: *"I fell down the steps and broke my neck. I don't care. I am old. It's time to go. It's all done..."*

Then Moira started talking about a beautiful place, the realm where souls are healed when a life ends. I refer to this place as the *"life between lives"*, a space where souls get healed after a life on earth. For me, this realm is where souls decide on a possible reincarnation and choose the lesson they want to learn in it. I know that there are fellow hypnotists, who specialize in successfully regressing clients to this out-of-earth life. I read about their amazing work and the effects these regressions have on their clients. I applaud them for their work and achievements.

Moira: *"I see angels. They are grabbing me by the arms and welcoming me. There is somebody above them... like a master. He has gold hair. He is smiling and says 'welcome'."*

BC: *"Do you remember what your lesson was in the lifetime as Marie?"*

Moira: *"Yes, it was helping others. I believe I fulfilled my lesson."*

BC: *"How do you feel leaving behind all the people you loved?"*

Moira: *"It was time. I will see them again..."*

How right she was, I thought to myself. Moira seemed sure that there is never a goodbye between our loved ones and us; it's only *"see you soon... in another life"*.

BC: *"Now I want you to go back to that lifetime as a little boy in a Slavic country. Remember that you were ten years old, in a house with a fireplace."*

Moira: *"I am still ten, standing in front of the fireplace looking at my dad. He swaps sides. Now he is on the right hand side. I've done something wrong. I will be told off. I remember... I left my little sister outside."*

BC: *"Who is your little sister?"*

Moira: *"I have two sisters: Lisa and Emily. They are twins."*

BC: *"Do you recognize them as being present in your current life?"*

Moira: *"Yes, they are two friends of mine now."*

BC: *"Move to another scene now, one that is relevant to you."*

Moira: *"I am walking outside the same house, but it's different. It is mine now. My parents are in the original part of the house. We built more and it has a proper roof now; it's bigger now. The old house is towards the back and the new extension at the front."*

BC: *"Do you remember how old you may be in this scene?"*

Moira: *"In my twenties. I have a girlfriend. We have baskets and we are going to the market with flowers."*

BC: *"Do you remember your name?"*

Moira: *"Jack again."*

BC: *"If nothing else happens, move in time to another scene in that existence."*

Moira: *"I am running a business. I am forty. People are coming and going... very successful... lots of barrels. I have a couple of kids running around. I have an older one, who runs the shop and two smaller ones... there is a bit of an age gap between them."*

BC: *"Tell me about your children."*

Moira: *"The boy who is taller than me is my son in the present. The little ones are five and six. I am very happy. Life is good."*

BC: *"Let's go to the moment of your death in the lifetime you revisited."*

Moira: *"I think I am on a ship going to Spain. I am going to buy new fabric. There is a storm. I am not going to make it. I die in the storm."*

BC: *"Who else dies with you?"*

Moira: *"Just about everyone on board. The sails came down. We were all trapped. My family is back home. My son will take over. He'll be fine..."*

BC: *"Is there any contract or promise you carried in the present?"*

Moira: *"Yes, I promised my family I would bring back new fabric, but I am not able to. They won't be able to expand. They will have to change plans. They will have to *go north to survive. Maybe they will have to do something else... something with oils. We talked about it. This is what they should do because I couldn't keep my promise."*

BC: *"Do you remember what the lesson was that you had to learn in this lifetime?"*

Moira: *"How to do things on my own. I learnt success. Just do it!"*

We spent a long time chatting after I brought Moira back to complete awareness and, while she shared more memories with me, I remembered how lucky I am, doing what I like most for a living. I love people and the connection I can establish with them it makes my life complete... especially when I regress a client like Moira, who is able to remember the incarnations of her loved ones in past lives. Each of the lifetimes she revisited brought back memories about people important to her in her current life and their experiences in the far past. There is hope that we never lose our loved ones and that death is just a bridge between lives. Every life is a miracle built around souls playing roles in each other's existences.

Nowadays we tend to associate success with fame. We live in weird times, when one is considered accomplished if she or he is cheered by the crowds; sometimes for no reason whatsoever. The more likes and followers one has on any of the social media networks, the more fame and ultimately fulfillment one gets. Success however has to do with the inner attainment we may achieve when we generate individual or collective progress. Success is a destination rather than a strategy; we reach it only if we follow a forward trajectory. In my opinion, success is a positive movement based on the desire - or even ambition - to make a positive change.

Just a few days ago, I was having coffee in a local cafe. Next to me, my beloved dog Hendrix enjoyed some deserved time away from home. As I tried focusing on my cup of coffee, a conversation between a woman and a man caught my attention. She, a mature beautiful woman, told him, probably her partner, *"you successfully destroyed our relationship"*. The sentence stayed with me for the whole day. On one hand I understood what the lady meant; on the other hand it seemed like utter nonsense. Success is a positive action towards a destination rather than a step backwards. There is no success in initiating destruction or a war; achievement is gained by installing peace, so as upset as the woman in the cafe might have been, her words made no sense. No one can have success in destroying; success goes with creation.

Moira's regression revealed another aspect regarding success. For her, providing for others and building an empire for her loved ones meant success. How would we know we have achieved fulfillment if there is nobody to experience it with us? We are part of universality and our success affects others. Therefore, going back to the couple debating in a cafe, success cannot - at least in my opinion - be based on hurting or destroying other people's feelings or lives. Fulfillment is just an ingredient much needed in reaching unconditional love.

From the early stages of our lives, we strive for success. We want to be somebody who achieves something. We set up year-by-year goals and we strategize to achieve them. Most people go even further and decide on New Year's resolutions. Our competitive nature pushes us higher and higher. *"People who succeed have momentum"*, said Tony Robbins; so aim to be the best version of yourself, one who can inspire other people to reach their maximum selves, because this excellence will help you achieve your personal success. And once you do that, you will constantly aim for it!.

Karmic lesson 3

FAMILY

"Life is about family"

The first thing I noticed about Tessa was her bubbly personality... and her beautiful skin. I thought to myself that people would pay heaps of money to have skin like hers. She didn't wear any make up when she turned up for her appointment and I tried not to stare at the perfect complexion of her skin.

    She started talking right after she sat down on the recliner in my practice and the conversation flowed beautifully. Some people are shy and feel it's more appropriate not to offer too much information about themselves; others prefer complete privacy when asked to share details about their lives. But not Tessa! She answered all my questions with open honesty. She talked about her responsibility as a single mother of two sons, her career as an early childhood teacher, her desire to find her soul mate someday, her garden and her property; in fact she told me exactly what I needed to know about her life... and even more. I admired her openness and wondered how was she able to fit in every chore and still be happy and content. At the end of the day, she was still very young, in her early thirties, and carrying so much weight on her shoulders.

Before even asking, Tessa said she felt that a past life regression would shine a little light on her busy current life. She may have been being honest again about the reason for the regression, but my thought was that it might also be her inclination for adventure, because Tessa liked to know and experience as much as she was able to... and I liked that about her!

Inducing trance was a breeze and I wished that I had more clients as determined to let themselves go as deeply as she did. Whilst guiding her to beaches and beautiful secluded gardens, I kept admiring her glowing olive skin that fitted perfectly with her light brown curly hair. Just behind her, I noticed the magnolias in my garden and that made me feel happy... as happy as Tessa was.

Tessa: *"It's one in the morning. It's dark. I am alone."*

BC: *"Can you see your feet even in this darkness?"*

Tessa: *"Yes... they are bigger... manly feet...no shoes..."*

BC: *"So you're a man. What are you wearing?"*

Tessa: *"Brown shorts, a brown vest and a white shirt. My feet are very dirty... I see the buttons of my vest. They look bluish."*

BC: *"What color is your hair?"*

Tessa: *"Short, dark blonde hair...and big blue eyes.... very light skin."*

BC: *"What else do you remember about yourself?"*

Tessa: *"My name is James. I am thirty-four."*

BC: *"Can you recall where you live?"*

Tessa: *"It's somewhere in England. I don't remember the county. The year is 1904."*

BC: *"Tell me what else you can see."*

Tessa: *"I see an old shed.... very old shed. I don't want to go into the shed. Something happened there...*

People got hurt in there. There are some people in blue uniform there... who hurt others."

BC: *"What do you know about those people?"*

Tessa: *"They wear blue uniforms with shiny buttons. They wear hats and have moustaches."*

BC: *"You don't like them..."*

Tessa: *"No. They are torturing people in there. They don't like us. They want our country. I can see one of them very well, but I don't think I know him."*

BC: *"What language do those people in blue uniform speak?"*

Tessa: *"Russian."*

BC: *"Now focus on your family. Do you have a wife and children?"*

Tessa: *"Yes, three children... two boys and a girl. They are four, five and nine years old."*

BC: *"Are any of your children people you know in your current life?"*

Tessa: *"One of them is my dad."*

BC: *"Do you have a wife?"*

Tessa: *"Yes, she is so pretty. Her name is Sally. She is my son now."*

BC: *"Tell me what happens in the shed."*

Tessa: *"There is an explosion.... big fire. I am outside the shed and feel the explosion. I see a man in blue uniform coming out another way. I don't recognize him, but he feels familiar. He is laughing."*

BC: *"As I count now from three to one, I want you to move to a significant scene in that lifetime as James. Where are you now?"*

As I started counting, my eyes were on Tessa. She looked young and beautiful. Behind her, in the garden, my black kitten Lily played silly games catching a butterfly.

Tessa: *"In a hole. I cannot get out. One of those men in blue uniforms locked me in. I am alone. I see the sky a little bit."*

BC: *"Why did he lock you in?"*

Tessa: *"They wanted my family. My family got pulled out of the house. They took them all, wife and children. They took them to the forest. They tied them up to the trees... they shot them. My family is not alive anymore."*

It is a humbling sensation to witness the pain of any of my clients when they recall sad memories. Therefore I felt Tessa's tenderness when talking about her family in a past life. Even sad, her skin was glowing and I felt a little envious.

BC: *"What happens next?"*

Tessa: *"I give up. I want to die."*

Tessa was silent for a few minutes before experiencing her death as James. She was wistful.

Tessa: *"I am still in that hole. I die of starvation."*

BC: *"Let your soul leave your body and tell me what you feel."*

Tessa: *"Life is about family and protecting your family. I didn't protect my family."*

BC: *"Don't worry about that. You've done your best. What else do you feel, see or hear?"*

Tessa: *"There is an angel next to me. I go with him. I am happy. I feel peaceful and healed now. I see my family. There is a dog there. I don't recognize him. He is brown with curly hair. I think that I had him when I was a young boy. His name is Chess."*

The subject about our pets in past lives, or in the life between lives, has never really been discussed in detail. Many people believe that animals go to a different place after death than humans do. I believe that we all depart to the same realm. Apparently Tessa shared my belief.

As there was nothing else she was willing to tell me about that lifetime as James, I decided that there was enough time to explore another life. Resilient, Tessa started remembering a totally different existence.

Tessa: *"I see stone walls and a castle. I am a young woman of nineteen. I have really long hair, plaited to my shoulders. I wear a white dress, a blue vest and red shoes."*

BC: *"Do you remember your name?"*

Tessa: *"My name is Gaby."*

BC: *"Where is the castle you were telling me about?"*

Tessa: *"In Scotland, in the 1700s. The castle belongs to my family. I have lots of money."*

BC: *"Are you in a relationship?"*

Tessa: *"Yes, with the prince. I don't trust him. All the girls like him. They flirt with him... He likes it."*

BC: *"Do you recognize him as being somebody you know in your present life?"*

Tessa: *"Not really."*

BC: *"So what happens next?"*

Tessa: *"I am inside now, at the table. There is so much food on the table. The prince is here with me. His family is here too. I am not married to him yet."*

BC: *"Move now to another scene in that lifetime; a scene that is more relevant to you."*

Tessa: *"He is leaving for somewhere. I don't know where he is going. His family goes with him. I am now married to him. We have twin boys. I am twenty-seven years old now."*

BC: *"Do you recognize the twins?"*

Tessa: *"One of them is my nana."*

BC: *"What happens next?"*

Tessa: *"He's gone. I am not happy he went away. I hope he comes back."*

BC: *"Pick now another memory in that lifetime. Is your husband back?"*

Tessa: *"No. He didn't want to come back. I grew old alone. I am eighty-nine years old. My children are with me. They have families now and I have grandchildren. They make me happy. I am dying of old age and my family is with me."*

BC: *"Let your soul leave the body. Can you recall what your lesson was in the lifetime you remembered?"*

Tessa: *"It's about family and being by myself. You can do it on your own. You can still be happy. I don't want to leave my boys. I made a promise to always be there for them."*

BC: *"It is the time now to break that promise. You don't have to prove anything anymore."*

Tessa: *"I can't leave my boys!"*

BC: *"Leave that promise in that lifetime and when you come back, come back without it. Break the promise."*

While Tessa became more aware and her beautiful face lightened up, I realized what a similarity there was between the lives she revisited and her current one. Tessa was all about family. She was a fighter, a woman capable of providing for her two sons no matter how hard that may have been. She was not a complainer and her intention of being regressed wasn't based on finding excuses for anything whatsoever. She didn't want to know if she carried responsibilities from past lives. She just wanted to know…

Tessa and I became even friendlier after the regression. As I suspected, she acknowledged that there are families and families…. and hers as a single mother of two children was just a normal brood. Time passed and she listed her home on the market and put an offer on another property, one that offered a bigger garden for her children. Typical Tessa… a fighter, a doer and a strong woman!

I often think that the responsibilities we have in a family cell are the hardest lessons to achieve in a lifetime. Society as a whole bases its structure on nuclear families; therefore evolution starts with the small cell we call family.

We are given people at our birth to look after and we chose people we want to take care of.

Family is a unit of socialization and it has its own particular and unique rules of cohabitation. As much as governments might intend to mandate, control or even ukase the family structure, they will be left disappointed, because the family unit defies any standard structure. The conservative layout of mother, father and children, each with archaic roles, described by the French sociologist Emile Durkheim, is no longer a standard, structured set-up in the twenty first century. No matter how a family functions and how duties are allocated, choosing people who serve our life paths and learning to coexist with them is still one of the hardest mission we, humans, are facing.

For Tessa, her children were in a past as well as in the present life her family, one that she protected, nurtured, loved and provided for; perhaps for others a partner, parents, or friends could be part of past and present lives. At the end of the day, living with others involves giving and receiving unconditional love, and we do that with the ones we chose to.

Karmic lesson 4

PATIENCE

"Wait and see how it turns out"

Sandra emailed me very early on a Sunday morning asking for an appointment, and I thought to myself how lucky this woman was, because I had a cancelation for the next day. Usually there is a waiting list and there is nothing I can do to help someone get in earlier. I replied straight away and Sandra confirmed her appointment in the next minute. I didn't know what to expect, nor had I guessed how old she may have been or why she wanted to be regressed.

She arrived the next day and, as I opened the door, I was surprised, if not shocked, to see that she had the most unusual and beautiful hair I have ever seen in my whole life: very long and curly, ginger-red color, somewhere in between an orange and a strawberry. *"It's my natural color"*, she said even before introducing herself. I couldn't stop looking at her amazing hair whilst thinking that women would pay a fortune to have hair like hers.

Sandra was a vision in white. On that fragile, gorgeous body, she wore a white lace summery dress and white sandals and to me she looked like a goddess. Even the way she walked was dreamy and I had the feeling that her feet barely touched the carpet. She seemed like she was floating.

In the long corridor, as we walked towards my practice, I asked her why she'd booked a past life regression. She took her time, sat down on the recliner in my practice and started talking with a soft voice, almost whispering about her life and why she thought that a regression session was needed. I could barely hear what she said, so I moved my chair closer to hers.

I let her talk for more than five minutes and realized that what she said made no sense. She jumped from one subject to another and I thought to myself that, perhaps because of her lack of confidence, she might have learnt by heart a variety of answers to my possible questions. So when she stopped for a second, I asked *"Now, very honestly, what is the reason you are here?"* She suddenly seemed to forget the answers she'd prepared in advance, dropped her mask, and said that she really wanted a child and now, that she was almost forty, the chances were getting slimmer and slimmer. I looked at her and couldn't believe what I heard. She looked like a young woman in her twenties!

I knew that she was being honest when she told me about her ex partners, none of whom wanted children. She thought that they all only wanted her, not the children she could have offered them. She said that at the present time she was in a complicated relationship with a man who, again, never talked about starting a family, and she had even been thinking of asking him to agree to have a child with her... and then leave after the birth. She wanted a child for herself! I understood that the relationship she was in was complicated all right, as she gave more details about it.

But as there was nothing else I needed to know about Sandra, I started making her more comfortable and relaxed and began inducing trance. She surrendered easily and embarked on our hypnotic conversation.

BC: *"Are you inside or outside?"*
Sandra: *"I am outside."*
BC: *"Look around. What do you see?"*
Sandra: *"Children. It's a city in England.... many children around."*
BC: *"Do you remember the year?"*
Sandra: *"1919."*
BC: *"Now look down at your feet. What are you wearing?"*
Sandra: *"I am barefoot. I wear a dress... light blue dress. I have black hair and green eyes."*

I wondered for a second if her hair was as unusual then as it was now, or if she looked as gorgeous then as now.

BC: *"Do you remember how old you are?"*
Sandra: *"I am thirty. My name is Samantha.... Yes, they call me Samantha."*
BC: *"Do you have any family?"*
Sandra: *"Yes, I am married to an unkind man. He has a top hat and a stick, maybe because he is limping. He doesn't have anything to do with me. We have lots of children together."*
BC: *"Tell me about the children."*
Sandra: *"I have seven children, four boys and three girls."*
BC: *"What else do you remember?"*
Sandra: *"I feel that I live in a big house, but I have to come to the village to do cleaning and washing clothes for others. I don't know what status I am, because I am poor, but I have a big house and I feel that I have no support from my husband, so I work my fingers to the bone. Whilst I work, the children are running around in the village."*

BC: *"Is your husband or are any of your children's energies familiar? Can you recognize any of them?"*

Sandra: *"My husband is one of my ex partners, and one of my children - a boy with dark hair - is my nephew now, who I have a strong bond with. This is my favorite child. His name is Andrew."*

BC: *"Why is he your favorite?"*

Sandra: *"Because he supports me. He is more like a friend and he helps me with the chores. He seems to care about my feelings."*

BC: *"Do you feel happy?"*

I asked the question, already knowing the answer, but I wanted her to express everything she might have felt in the past life she had decided to revisit.

Sandra: *"No. My partner is not there for me and I have to look after my children. It's hard!"*

BC: *"Why did you marry him?"*

Sandra: *"Through association.... procedures that I had to do... yes, I had to."*

BC: *"Are your parents alive?"*

Sandra: *"Yes, they are."*

BC: *"What is your relationship with them?"*

Sandra: *"My mother lets me do writing at a desk when I visit her. I like writing my thoughts down. There are flowers in a jar on the desk. The window is open... My mother is gentle with me."*

BC: *"Do you recognize her energy?"*

Sandra: *"She is my grandmother."*

BC: *"I will now count from three to one and I want you to go a year further in time and see what happens."*

I started counting down, and then waited for Sandra to share more with me. Her face was glowing and her beautiful hair looked even shinier. I had no clue why I thought of my hairdresser's salon back in Auckland at that moment, but I knew that she would have loved the challenge of reproducing a hair color like Sandra's.

Sandra: *"I am sitting at a table. I wear a white shirt with a nice collar around the neck. I am at the dinner table with my husband and our children."*

BC: *"What is the relationship with him now?"*

Sandra: *"He is nice. He changed. We are at the dinner table and he talks to me and we laugh. He is involved in my energy."*

BC: *"Involved?"*

Sandra: *"Yes, because I am happier now. We are laughing a lot. He is funny and there is no hassle anymore. We have enough money. I am not serving him as I was before... we are friends and lovers now."*

BC: *"Tell me about the children."*

Sandra: *"Andrew is cheeky and funny. He is so happy... He is enjoying his academic work. He has a good brain. He's lost that sadness... he is happy that he has a mom and a dad."*

BC: *"That's nice. Move now to another moment in that lifetime and, when you are there, tell me what you see, hear or feel."*

Sandra: *"I am forty-one years old now. I am in the forest or maybe in a park with my family. We are having a picnic. My husband is sitting down on the blanket with us and he is so nice... He is not demanding. Our children are enjoying the day out."*

BC: *"How is Andrew doing?"*

Sandra: *"Just before... he was sitting relaxed with us... now he's standing up. He is a good boy. He studies Agriculture at university."*

BC: *"Can you remember your surname?"*

Sandra: *"Satchi. My name is Samantha Satchi."*

Sandra was my first client who remembered her surname in a past life and to be perfectly honest, when I asked for it, I didn't expect her to recall it. However her answer came quickly and she seemed very sure about her surname. In past life regressions, there is always a first and my clients never stop surprising me with the variety of detailed memories they can bring forward.

BC: *"Do you feel that there was any contract or promise you made in that lifetime?"*

Sandra: *"I think there was something between my dad and this man he married me off to... something involving me. It was an arrangement I wasn't happy about. But then, we became friends and lovers. At the beginning I felt that I wasn't a real human because it was a business arrangement."*

BC: *"If you still feel uncomfortable with that contract and the sadness that brought with it at the beginning of your marriage, all you have to do is to break it. Therefore coming back into the present you can leave any residual energy behind."*

Then Sandra recalled the moment of her death in the lifetime that started in the early 1900s in England. She felt that it wasn't long after the picnic scene in the park when she got sick and died of something related to her lungs. She seemed relieved that her children were old enough to take care of themselves. So I asked if she remembered the lesson learnt in that past life.

Sandra: *"Patience. Wait and see how it turns out. People change."*

Sandra and I talked for another half an hour after the session. *"To be honest, I just wanted to know if I ever had children... and now I know"*, she said, emphasizing the fact that deep down she always thought that she had been a mother once. She admitted that her desire to bring life to the world was still there, but she decided to follow what Samantha Satchi taught her in a long lost life: *"wait and see how it turns out"*.

I haven't seen Sandra since the regression, but we are now friends on social media and I read her posts with great interest. None of them revealed any baby news though and none of them revealed a partner. I often wonder whether she found peace with the partner she was involved with when I first met her, or if she let him go. But no matter how she decided to live her life, Sandra proved to me that sometimes we are given what we want and other times our prayers are unanswered by the mighty Universe. I am not sure why this may happen but I know precisely that, whatever our life paths may be, we are all aiming towards perfection.

We sometimes face delays in achieving the state of inner peace and happiness we desire. There may be moments when we reach crossroads or feel stuck; there may be blockages that stop up reaching goals. At all these times, forbearance is required. It is not a case of waiting for miracles to happen; it is about manifesting what we desire to happen and deciding on our actions whilst waiting.

Cognitive neuroscience recognizes patience as part of the decision making process, whilst in the main religious dogmas it may have totally different connotations. In Buddhism for instance, patience is one of the *"perfections"*, whilst for Hinduism it is the main virtue. The same value is recognized by Christianity and Islam as a virtue. The German philosopher Friedrich Nietzsche however argued that only *"passion will not wait"*.

Patience is a characteristic of wise people. They know that things happen in a natural order, dictated by circumstances and situations. *"All in good time"*, as the Roman poet and philosopher Horace said.

No matter how much effort I put into researching karma, I have never come across patience as being a karmic lesson, so Sandra's past life regression taught me that we may have to hold back wishing for favorable things to happen and good people to come our way. Nobody is waiting for a catastrophe.

Patience requires extra virtues such as self-control, perseverance, tolerance and endurance; all of them part of our physical, emotional, mental and spiritual development and evolvement. So, once we learn to wait, we may be a step closer to finding inner peace.

Karmic lesson 5

TRUST

"You have to help yourself first"

Simon was one of the first people I met when I moved to this new city a few years ago and, since then, he has had a few past life regressions with me. He was one of the cases I described in my first book *"You have lived many times"*. As an energy healer, he is miraculous; as a person he is awesome. I am a big fan of his work and he values mine. It's a win-win situation.

Simon is a gentle bear and everybody likes him. He is soft, kind and empathetic. He always has a wise word for everybody and he puts all his efforts into helping others. I like everything about him, including his friendly partner, Fay. Together they are invincible.

Early this year, Simon had a weird accident that caused ligaments and tendons ruptures in his left arm, just above the wrist. After being in a cast for a while, he had to go through surgery. Right after being discharged from the hospital, Simon called and booked in for another past life regression. I have to admit that I was delighted to guide him through another regression, as I found his memories in the past quite fascinating.

He came in with his partner and after chatting for a while, he admitted that he was having a few recurring dreams lately that sometimes ended up in nightmares. I thought to myself that, with his calm and positive nature, he should be the last person to have nightmares. I imagined that the boredom of not being able to work because of the injury was to blame, but he believed that all his recent dreams were initiated by releasing something from his past lives.

Without any other comment, I started his new journey into his past. Inducing hypnosis was a breeze because, as I have said, Simon had already been through some hypnosis sessions with me and was able to surrender easily. Therefore, just a few minutes later, I was able to start asking questions.

BC: *"Can you see your feet?"*

Simon: *"Only just. My feet are bigger. I am a cowgirl. I've got cowboy boots on."*

BC: *"Can you see the color of your boots?"*

Simon: *"Tan, dusty with spears on the back."*

BC: *"What about your hands?"*

Simon: *"I have working hands... big."*

BC: *"What are you wearing?"*

Simon: *"A dress... that is not like a dress... it looks different... It's whitish color... dusty."*

BC: *"What else can you remember about yourself?"*

Simon: *"My long hair is wavy and curly... light brown. My eyes are light blue. I have olive skin."*

BC: *"Can you remember how old you are?"*

Simon: *"I am in my twenties."*

BC: *"What is your name?"*

Simon: *"Sophia.... Sophia Thompson."*

Not many people are able to remember in a past life regression their surnames, but Simon was a man of many details. Just a few weeks before him, Sandra recalled her surname too. Nothing surprises me anymore when I conduct regressions. Some clients recall details in a pedantic manner; others are more general.

BC: *"Where are you at the moment?"*

Simon: *"In a ranch in Texas."*

BC: *"What year is it?"*

Simon: *"In the 1820s."*

BC: *"Do you have any family?"*

Simon: *"Yes... sisters and brothers... big family."*

BC: *"Do you get along with everybody?"*

Simon. *"Half pie I mainly get along with my dad. Some of my brothers like me, others don't. I can outgun them."*

BC: *"What is your dad's name?"*

Simon: *"Jonathan."*

BC: *"Do you remember your mother?"*

Simon: *"Yes. She is always cooking. Her name is Dorothy."*

BC: *"Were your parents born in Texas?"*

Simon: *"My mother was. My father came from overseas. He was born in Ireland."*

BC: *"Do you have a boyfriend?"*

Simon: *"No. Men don't like me because I have power. I am strong. And I can read and write... that's why they don't like me."*

BC: *"Tell me more about that ranch."*

Simon: *"It's huge... huge. Lots of cattle... I don't see my neighbors much because they live far away. The house is nice and loving."*

BC: *"So what are you doing now?"* Simon: *"At the moment, nothing... I am just kicking dust around."*

It wasn't in Simon's nature to be cheeky, so I enjoyed this side to him.

BC: *"So what do you like doing?"*

Simon: *"Riding horses and shooting. I have my own horse. It's light tan with a white patch."*

BC: *"Is this a happy life?"*

Simon: *"It's a very good life."*

I instructed Simon to move to another scene in the life as Sophia and waited for a few minutes until he was ready to share more memories with me.

Simon: *"I am very old... eighty something. I am still on the ranch... sitting on the porch... waiting for dinner to be cooked. One of my daughters cooks."*

Simon mentioned children for the first time so I assumed that Sophia might have been married. A past life regression session is a creative protocol; therefore everything a client may say opens up a new chapter in remembering, only if the therapist really listens to what is being said. And I do; so I decided to find out more about Sophia's family, living in a ranch, in Texas.

BC: *"Did you have a man in your life?"*

Simon: *"Yes, I was married. My husband died. I have a big family."*

BC: *"What was his name?"*

Simon: *"John."*

BC: *"I want you now to go back in time and remember how you met John."*

Simon: *"We met horse riding. He came around traveling. He was born in the area."*

BC: *"Did you like him straight away?"*

Simon: *"No, we argued... Then we spent time together..."*

BC: *"Do you remember your wedding?"*

Simon: *"Yes, it was awesome. Many people..."*

BC: *"Are any of those people somebody you know in the present life?"*

Simon: *"One of my neighbors is my mother now."*

BC: *"How many children do you have?"*

Simon: *"Oh, we have a big family... boys and girls."*

BC: *"Are any of your children somebody in your life now?"*

Simon: *"My youngest boy is my partner Fay. His name is Tom."*

BC: *"What is your relationship with Tom?"*

Simon: *"Pretty good. He is the youngest. He gets on with a lot."*

BC: *"Is he going to take over the ranch?"*

Simon: *"I don't know... probably he will..."*

BC: *"Tell me how did John die."*

Simon: *"Some said it was the horse... some said he was shot."*

BC: *"And what do you believe?"*

Simon: *"I think he got shot."*

BC: *"Do you or your children know who shot him?"*

Simon: *"We don't know. I think it was somebody who wanted maybe to pinch our cattle."*

BC: *"So now you are old and John is not around anymore. Who will take over the ranch?"*

Simon: *"My children... it's a family thing. They all work together. All my kids are good."*

BC: *"Move now to the last moments in this lifetime. Where are you?"*

Simon: *"Sitting on my porch. I am still in my eighties. I am dying in my sleep. My family is watching me."*

BC: *"What was the lesson you learnt in this life?"*

Mike: *"Survive... trust in being yourself."*

I have always enjoyed the amount of detail Simon remembered from his past lives. So I decided to keep this session going for as long as time permitted. I asked him to revisit another life and he jumped instantly into another body.

Simon: *"I am in a jazz club in New Orleans. I am playing the saxophone... at this jazz festival. We've got an awesome band. We just tour around and play jazz. There is a bus waiting for us."*

BC: *"Is there anybody you recognize in your band?"*
Simon: *"Yes, my brother now."*
BC: *"What do you remember about yourself?"*
Simon: *"I am a black man in my fifties."*
BC: *"What are you wearing?"*
Simon: *"Shiny black shoes and a suit."*
BC: *"Can you remember your name?"*
Simon: *"My name is Sam."*
BC: *"Do you remember the year?"*
Simon: *"Early 1900s."*
BC: *"Do you have any family?"*
Simon: *"Nah... I am always on the road."*
BC: *"Was there a woman for you in the past?"*
Simon: *"There was the girl of my dreams, a white girl. Her name was Samantha. I didn't marry her because her father didn't let us. He was a wealthy racist man. He was in the air force. We had words and he told me I wasn't allowed to see his daughter. Samantha cried... Then they moved away and I never saw them again. I don't know where they moved. I never met another woman."*
BC: *"Is he somebody you recognize?"*
Mike: *"Yes, he is my uncle now."*

I started counting down and guided Simon to the last minutes of the lifetime as Sam, a jazz saxophone player in New Orleans.

Simon: *"I am on a bus. I am in my sixties. We have a new driver. The bus goes off the cliff and most of us die."*
BC: *"What was the lesson you learnt as Sam?"*
Mike: *"Trust that you survive."*

I looked at the huge clock on the wall and realized that I was able to squeeze in another few minutes, so I let Simon decide whether or not he wanted to revisit a different past life. He started talking instantly.

Simon: *"I am in house... in a lounge. There is a couch, a TV and many toys. I am one or two years old. I wear diapers and a shirt."*

BC: *"Tell me about your parents."*

Simon: *"They love me. My mother has black, curly hair and my father's hair is black and very short. My mother looks after me and my father is selling things. I don't have any brothers."*

BC: *"What do you remember about yourself?"*

Simon: *"My hair is blondish and my eyes blue. I don't remember my name."*

BC: *"That's fine. You may remember it later. Go now to another scene in the same lifetime."*

Simon: *"I am in a park in New York. It's the early 1960s. I see bushes. I am three years old. There are people around. I am happy... I remember my name now. It's Nicky."*

BC: *"Is there anybody you recognize in the present life?"*

Simon: *"Yes, there is that boy in my neighborhood. He is Fay now."*

Then Simon remembered another memory, this time closer to the moment of death.

Simon: *"I am five. There's fire everywhere... electrical fault. I am trapped. I can't see my parents, but I know they are in the house. They cannot get to me. I am scared. I see the ceiling falling down. I know I'm going to die."*

BC: *"Do you?"*

Simon: *"Yes. As I die, I can see from above the house burning down and my mom and dad crying. I hear voices telling me 'welcome home'. There are heaps of spirits there... family, friends, and buddies. I love it here. I don't want to go back."*

I realized that Simon's soul left the body of the little five year old boy and went to a place we call *"life between lives"*. As I mentioned before, I resume my sessions to memories from past lives only, giving my clients the option of sharing memories from this special realm, or not. In my experience, all my clients were able to see their souls leaving their bodies, but only some had memories from in between incarnations. Simon was one of them.

BC: *"Do you remember what lesson you had to learn in this short life?"*

Simon: *"Yes. Trust that... people have to help people."*

BC: *"Is there anything else you see or hear?"*

Simon: *"I am being told by angels that we have to figure things out. They help you achieve your mission, but you have to help yourself first."*

While Simon opened his eyes, my thoughts went to what just happened. I was wondering how revisiting these lives would help him understand the cause, or message of his recurring dreams. But Simon wasn't confused at all. What he took from the past lives he recalled was that he had to trust the whole process of recovering. Perhaps the Universe had a plan for him, bigger that he could see, and his injury was part of it.

It was the next day when I got a message from Simon. I smiled as I opened it. He wanted to let me know that after the regression, just on the way back home, he remembered clearly how the fire started. He said that, when he was five as Nicky, he already had a baby brother. He recalled how his brother crawled on the floor and how he tripped over him and hit something that started the fire. Sometimes clients remember even more in the first forty-eight hours after the regression.

When we refer to trust, we usually mean relying on somebody in order to achieve something. Not many, however, ponder that we have to first lean on our own abilities to survive and perhaps then reach our desires.

Trust is frequently referred to our relationships with others; or with our own internal beliefs as inner self-trust; whilst faith is the equivalent of trust in the conviction of a higher energy - referred to as God. For me, trust is what frees us from the fear of not fitting in. As much as we desire to trust ourselves and others, when we sense that we don't belong in a situation or don't appertain to a group, we fear; and the more we lose control, the lower the sense of trust goes.

Trust is a logical act; we can choose to trust others and ourselves, or we can decide to doubt. It is also an emotion that cannot be summoned on demand. We cannot ask others to be reliable enough for us to trust them; whether we do or we don't trust them is totally up to us. Therefore trust is not a reciprocal equation. We can instill it by being genuine, but we cannot expect one to prove their trust to us.

Some say that we only trust people we love. I am not sure this is always the case. We don't necessarily have to love somebody to believe that his or her acts are legitimate. In saying that, would we trust our lives to people we don't love? We build up trust and we break trust. We don't trust at first sight though; we need proof that we can confide in somebody.

In my opinion, we trust the virtual world of the Internet more than the people we know. We share online not just our personal details, but we also give out our darkest secrets. We trust millions of people whom we know nothing about and - in our naivety - we believe that they are our friends who care. We trust them more than others because we are desperately seeking love and approval and we are not suspicious for a second that our details could be used against us. We have trust issues with our loved ones when they make the smallest accidental mistakes, but we don't have any trust problems with the rest of the whole world.

A few days ago, I was watching a reality show on TV, one of the very popular ones in my country. There, a group of twelve beautiful girls were fighting with each other in the hope that they would win the heart of a single guy, who to be honest, was far from worth fighting over. Each of the contestants tried to hide aspects of their lives, not trusting the others with sharing things that would make them look less perfect. However, they trusted the network to reveal to millions of people everything about them. That made me think that we often don't trust people we know and trust the ones we don't. But, in saying that, society changes, and with it, we change too. Whatever was relevant yesterday may not be relevant today.

Karmic lesson 6

EMPATHY

"Don't be an arse"

My phone rang one Friday around lunchtime and I heard a strong voice introducing herself as Joyce and asking for a booking. Even before I asked what the reason was for the regression session, Joyce said, *"something is holding me back and I have to know why"*. Good enough motive for me, I thought to myself. I made the booking and right after hanging up I realized that the whole phone conversation lasted for less than a minute. Usually, when clients call me, they find it necessary to elaborate in detail on their lives; but not Joyce. I already felt that she may be the perfect client... and my intuition was spot on.

The first thing I noticed about Joyce when she arrived for her appointment was that she was a very dynamic woman, always on the move, always doing something, constantly arranging her hair, her blouse or even making sure that her handbag was perfectly straight on the chair next to her. She came in early and answered straight to the point to all my questions. No metaphors, no long descriptions; just pure facts.

From what she said about herself, I figured out that Joyce was a hard working lady. For a person who worked her whole life for over sixty hours a week, she should have built up a fortune... but she hadn't. Never putting herself first, Joyce enjoyed helping out her adult son, her friends and neighbors. It was never about her and being the strong shoulder for everybody's problems was what she enjoyed most. However, lately she'd started feeling annoyed about the fact that her life was all work and no play. She perhaps realized that she was the only one in charge of her own happiness, and her busy schedule left almost no time for enjoyment and fun.

Recently separated from a long term relationship, Joyce decided that she didn't need another partner to make her happy, but her plan hadn't worked out because she still wasn't having any fun in her life.

Joyce's body relaxed immediately after I started taking her to the enigmatic world of hypnosis. Whilst talking about secluded gardens, I noticed more things about her, which I hadn't seen when she first came in. In her late forties, Joyce had strong muscles that reminded me of wild Mongol horses. For a woman of medium height, she had very long, beautiful legs with strong calves; and her face, with powerful jaws and prominent cheekbones, showed determination. I knew that she badly wanted to surrender to the whole process and find her answers, so, she let herself go very fast.

Once in trance, she answered my questions in a cheeky manner with a slight smile at the corner of her mouth. For a moment I thought to myself that she was amazed that she could see her past life so clearly.

Joyce: *"I feel like I am in space somewhere, maybe on the moon. It definitely looks like the moon. I feel safe though... no alarm bells."*

BC: *"Just take your time and land in a scene where you can feel, hear or see. Let me know when you are there."*

Joyce: *"I see my feet.... they look like they have white boots on them... not big feet. I've got nothing on my legs. Just bare skin... quite pale skin. I wear shorts and a red T-shirt."*

BC: *"How old are you?"*

Joyce: *"I am a teenager... I am thirteen. I am in no man's land. I am wandering around like I am lost. Somebody put me here."*

The first thing that came to my mind was that perhaps the lifetime Joyce decided to revisit might have finished when she was thirteen and all I wanted to know was what might have happened. I therefore decided to start her past life from the beginning with the earliest memory she was able to recall.

BC: *"No problem. Maybe go back in time to a scene when you were younger."*

Joyce: *"I am about three or four. I am crying lots. I am on the floor somewhere. I can see a bench and on the other side of the bench is my mother. She is medium build, brownish hair. She ignores me. I don't think that she loves me a lot. She doesn't hate me, but... She is just there."*

BC: *"Do you recognize her energy as being somebody in the present life?"*

Joyce: *"Yes, she is my grandmother. My mother's mother."*

BC: *"Do you have any siblings?"*

Joyce: *"No, I am the only child. I am a girl. My name is Janice."*

BC: *"Is your father around?"*

Joyce: *"No, he is not. He is working. He is doing trades... selling... buying..."*

BC: *"Tell me more about your home."*

Joyce: *"I see old furniture. I am in the lounge, on the floor and I see old pieces of furniture."*

BC: *"I want you to move in time to another scene in that lifetime as Janice. And when you are there, tell me what you see, hear or feel."*

Joyce: *"I am ten years old. I am on a horse... brown horse. I am in a big green paddock. I feel that I am in New Zealand because it looks very green. I can see some big pine trees on my right. I feel happy."*

BC: *"Go just a little bit further in time. Maybe another year."*

Joyce: *"I am eleven years old and I spend all my time with my horse. It makes me happy. My father is never around... He is a working man."*

BC: *"Do you recognize him as being somebody in the current life?"*

Joyce: *"The feeling I have is the feeling I have about my father."*

Joyce's father died a few years ago and she mentioned him before the regression. She told me that they have been very close and that she never totally recovered after he passed away.

BC: *"Move now back to the age of thirteen years old as I count from one to three."*

I waited for a few minutes for Joyce to get into the scene that her subconscious had chosen to revisit. The smile on her face disappeared suddenly.

Joyce: *"I am thinking about boys now and the horse takes second place. I am in a big school hall with loads of people in it... many children and adults. Everyone is in the school; many children in school uniform just chatting. I don't feel comfortable; I don't like it. I don't know why, but I don't like it."*

BC: *"Just move another month forward in time. Find yourself a month later."*

Joyce: *"I see an old farm house on a long driveway. There are people in the house, but I don't know who."*

BC: *"Go closer to the house and look in the window."*

Joyce: *"It's my family just ready to have dinner. I am outside. I don't want to go inside. I don't know why. I feel OK, but I don't want to be with them. They don't call me in. I don't even know if they care I am not there. I am wandering outside."*

BC: *"If you feel comfortable, move another few minutes later."*

Joyce: *"I am in a dark place. I don't remember how I got there and I don't know why I am there. I don't like the dark. It is cold. Temperature is cooler. I am alone."*

I tried understanding how she got to that dark place and what exactly might have happened. All Joyce remembered was that her life finished then. She said that she was outside her house and somebody dragged her somewhere. I figured out that there was no chance of her recalling anything else from that lifetime, so I decided to let her choose to reveal another incarnation.

BC: *"Now, I want you to move to a scene in another life. It's up to you which."*

Joyce started instantly remembering memories from another of her soul's existences.

Joyce: *"I am in a totally different world in some town and I see dusty roads where you can tie horses up. I am ten. I thought I was older but I am only ten. I wear jeans and a little vest. I am a boy."*

BC: *"Where are your parents?"*

JM: *"They have been killed."*

BC: *"So, can you remember who looks after you?"*

Joyce: *"I have the feeling that my grandmother is taking care of me..."*

BC: *"What can you remember about her?"*

Joyce: *"She has a bun in her hair... she is kind."*

BC: *"What is your name?"*
Joyce: *"Tommy. They call me Tommy."*
BC: *"Do you remember the year?"*
Joyce: *"Precisely. It's 1863."*
BC: *"What about the country?"*
Joyce: *"I remember it is Brazil."*
BC: *"Move now a few years later as Tommy."*
Joyce: *"I am in lots of trouble. Tommy has gone off the rails. I am causing trouble. I am seventeen and I play a lot with my guns... just being an arse"*
BC: *"Is your grandmother still alive?"*
Joyce: *"Yes. She still has the bun in her hair."*
BC: *"Jump now to another significant scene and tell me what you see."*
Joyce: *"I am twenty-five now. I've just been shot. I annoyed so many people. It's daytime and I am lying on the ground... in the streets. A guy shot me."*
BC: *"Try to identify him. Look into his eyes. Can you recognize him?"*
Joyce: *"Oh, my God! My father shot me... my father!"*

I knew that Joyce recognized the energy of her father in the present lifetime and that came as a surprise to her.

BC: *"Tell me what you see. Maybe float above your body whilst looking down to the street. What do you see?"*
Joyce: *"I am not ready to die. I am just lying there. No one is doing anything. They are just looking at me. Some say that I got what I deserved. I feel that one of them is one of my half brothers now. No one helps. I see my whole life in front of my eyes."*
BC: *"Do you remember your lesson in that life?"*
Joyce: *"Empathy. Don't be an arse. I had a choice but I didn't know how to live."*
BC: *"Look at the person who shot you. How do you feel about him?"*

Joyce: *"I don't feel anything... just pain... He feels remorse, but he had to do it."*

BC: *"What else do you remember about Tommy and that lifetime?"*

Joyce: *"I wasn't handsome. I had acne on my face. I never had a girlfriend. I was a loner. I didn't like people and people didn't like me."*

Once aware, Joyce seemed at peace with the memories she recalled in her past lives. Sometimes it may be difficult to believe that clients could uncover mysteries in the present life just by revisiting past ones... but they do and this makes my work even more exciting. Joyce seemed to believe that she had proof that she hadn't learnt what empathy was in the life as Tommy, and that her soul may have decided to reincarnate in the present only to understand and fulfill the lesson of sharing compassion and love with others. I wasn't sure that this was the case but, at the end of the day, my clients have to figure things out for themselves.

Empathy, along with love, is what keeps us, humans, together, but in most cases it is easier to love than to identify and experience someone else's feelings. In day-to-day life, we continuously try to be aware of our own inner self and the emotional response to everything that is outside us, or may not concern us, in a certain moment. We crave the sympathy of people, but we are not always ready to be empathetic to them.

Empathy, for me, means putting yourself in other people's shoes, understanding where they come from and accepting where they are going. It is a sentiment based on comprehending social differences and recognizing the way others feel and express emotions. Therefore, empathy may be even harder to achieve than sympathy and compassion. Being sympathetic to what others experience doesn't necessarily mean that we can identify ourselves as going through the same things as that person. Being empathetic, however, comprises leaving behind our point of view, tolerating and accepting other peoples' perspective by placing ourselves in the same situation.

Sometimes, our pets are more empathetic than we are. They sense when we suffer, are in pain or in danger and they feel when we are happy. They mimic our emotions by making them theirs. You may argue that this comes from the love they express to us; but what about an animal's reaction to another animal in sufferance when they see it for the first time?

Empathy is a primary feeling we may or may not be born with and develops as we grow. If love can make this planet a better place, empathy would definitely keep it that way forever.

Karmic lesson 7

INTEGRITY

"Stay true to yourself"

As a professional, I should not have favorites, but I do. Don't get me wrong. Every client gets the same treatment... except James. He is a little bit special. Maybe it is the fact that he is British like my husband; or perhaps that he thinks and acts in a very similar way to him.

I met James last year when he had a first past life regression with me. I presented his case in my book *"You have lived many times"*. Since then, he has attended a group regression I organized in one of the local centers and I also treated him using traditional hypnotherapy. James and I kept in touch during that whole time. We are both the kind of people who text each other when they have something to say and don't bother when they don't.

James is a very smart guy, who understands that a dream starts with a dreamer. He is exactly what we all aim to be: soft but strong, funny but serious, introvert but way out there, smart but humble, excited but relaxed. On top of that, James is a spiritual being who I love learning from. He, like me, doesn't take spirituality to the level where it becomes more like a cult than a way of living. Actually, we recently talked about the fact that we don't believe in anything in particular, but we are open to everything. Did I mention that he is also a drummer like me?

James arrived early evening one Friday. He was my last client for the day and I was looking forward my first weekend off in quite a while. Just before he parked his car, I inspected my rose bushes that were blooming crazily like never before. It's easy being happy when nature is.

As I have said, I enjoy talking with James because there is always something new I can learn from him. I just hope that this is reciprocal. Therefore we chatted for a while about the latest books we'd read and new things that impressed us in everyday life. Then I began the induction. I knew that James would go under fast and hoped he would revisit amazing lives.

BC: *"Tell me what you see, hear or feel."*

James: *"I am a man. I am wearing expensive shiny black shoes and a dark color suit I think."*

BC: *"How old are you?"*

James: *"Almost thirty."*

BC: *"Do you wear any ring or watch?"*

James: *"Yes, I have a wedding ring."*

BC: *"So you are married. What can you remember about your wife?"*

James: *"Her name is Alice. She has black hair... same age as me... Very pretty, very smiley. We don't have children yet."*

BC: *"Can you remember your name?"*

James: *"My name is Francis."*

BC: *"Look around. What can you see?"*

James: *"I am outdoors. It's raining. I have an umbrella. I am on the streets... it feels like an American street... big city... New York. There are many people around. It's busy. Even though it's raining, I am immaculately presented."*

BC: *"Were you born in that city?"*

James: *"I was born here, but Alice came from overseas... from England."*

BC: *"What year is it?"*

James: *"1917."*

BC: *"What are you doing for a living?"*

James: *"I am a banker... a senior partner. Yes, on the board of a bank."*

BC: *"What about Alice? Does she work?"*

James: *"No, she is at home keeping everything running well."*

BC: *"Now focus on Alice. Do you remember her as being somebody in the present life?"*

James surprised me when he answered. Usually clients recognize the energy of people involved in past lives as of somebody in their current life. James though remembered differently. He was the first client who referred to what we call the division of souls, in which one soul divides at some stage in two or more souls.

James: *"I do, but she seems like a mixture of several people: two of my friends and my sister...all together... in one person."*

BC: *"So you are walking on the street. Do you know where you are going?"*

James: *"I think I am still at work... I am going to a meeting."*

BC: *"Tell me what happens next."*

James: *"I am going up the steps of a large building. It looks like a hotel. People at reception seem to know who I am. I've been shown the way to a very posh lounge-bar area. There is a man sitting at a table with a long cigar in his hand. He is waiting for me. He has a long beard."*

BC: *"So you came to meet up with this man."*

James: *"Yes. His name is Edgar. We do business together. He works in the printing industry. He's got something for me to sign. We both sign the papers."*

BC: *"Do you recognize him as somebody you know in your present life?"*

James: *"Yes. He is a friend now."*

BC: *"Now look at the papers you signed. What are they?"*

James: *"There is a seal. It looks like a contract... although it looks like a loan agreement. The bank is lending him money."*

BC: *"Do you see the name or logo of the hotel?"*

James: *"I see a laurel leaf in a circle and the letter 'H'."*

As he described the hotel's logo, I knew exactly which one it was because my great grandmother spent a long time there and she kept some serviettes as a memory of that place. I saw them as a little girl and later in life I tried finding more details about that hotel in New York. Unfortunately, it was later renamed once it changed ownership. I couldn't say I wasn't surprised about James' memory - because I was - but most of all I was pleased that James had been there just a few years earlier than my great grandmother.

BC: *"Move now to another scene that is relevant to you."*

James: *"I am at home. It's massive. I am in my study. I see my desk and my bookshelf, full of books. There is a window, a little balcony and the view of some gardens. Alice is not with me in the room. She may be out somewhere."*

BC: *"How old are you now?"*

James: *"Older... maybe in my sixties."*

BC: *"Still no children?"*

James: *"There is a picture on the wall of a young girl. I think she may be adopted. She looks Latin American... dark hair, dark skin. She is not a child of ours. Her name is Maria. I remember that she is at university. Very clever girl..."*

BC: *"Is she somebody you know in the present life?"*

James: *"Yes, she is one of my friends now."*

BC: *"How is the business going?"*

James: *"I think I might have retired. Money is not an object. I see that Alice is here now. She is wearing a long dress, very immaculate dress. Very well presented. She is happy. We get along very well. She started painting recently."*

BC: *"So what happens?"*

James: *"Alice comes to get me. She tells me that I am retired so I don't need to work. So we take a walk in the garden. Many people are working in the garden."*

BC: *"Go now to the last moments in the live you revisited."*

James: *"It's dark. I can't see. I think that I am blind. I am old. I believe that I am in a therapy room. I am dying of old age."*

BC: *"Is Alice still around?"*

James: *"Yes. She is doing well. Maria is well also. She's got a husband and a child, a young girl."*

BC: *"What did you learn in the life as Francis?"*

James: *"Integrity."*

I looked at James as he remembered the mission he had to accomplish in the past life as a wealthy banker and realized that his life in the present was also an existence based on integrity. Is it possible for one to carry the virtues accumulated in past lives? Buddhism bases its doctrine on the fact that lessons are not passed from one life to another, but what if they are? While James remained relaxed on the recliner, my mind wandered, thinking about various religions and their approaches to reincarnation. Without making any judgment about one being better than another, I then guided James to a different past life.

James: *"I am on the beach with friends. I am a twenty year old woman. I wear a red and white swimming suit."*

BC: *"What else do you remember about yourself?"*

James: *"I have dark hair and brown eyes. My name is Aisha."*

BC: *"Do you know where that beach is?"*

James: *"It's hot... white sand. It's a big island. We speak Spanish."*

BC: *"What is the year?"*

James: *"1952."*

James kept silent for a while, so I knew that it was time to ask him to revisit another memory in the same lifetime.

James: *"I am in a very small apartment. I am a housekeeper. I may be twenty-four now."*

BC: *"So what happens in that apartment?"*

James: *"There is shouting down in the street."*

BC: *"Can you look out the window?"*

James: *"Yes. Someone I know is having an argument. It's a friend I am fond of, I guess. It turns into a fight. I run down the stairs and when I get there I see that my friend got hit. He is not moving. There is blood... and there are people who help me. I'm just hysterically crying. The other guy ran away."*

BC: *"Is your friend dead?"*

James: *"He must be... he is not moving."*

BC: *"Do you recognize any of those people?"*

James: *"Some of them. I recognize my friend who died. He is a friend now."*

BC: *"Leave this memory behind and move to the last minutes in this lifetime as Aisha."*

James: *"It's just a few weeks later... same year... I am on a bridge... falling off... I jumped."*

BC: *"Why?"*

James: *"I couldn't forget my friend. As I am falling down I am thinking of him too."*

BC: *"Any messages you may hear whilst falling?"*

James: *"Opportunity missed... stay true to yourself! Don't miss opportunities!"*

James opened his eyes and waited a while before he spoke again. It was almost dark in my practice and my thoughts flew to the weekend... my first weekend off in quite a while. I looked out of the window and noticed the red leaves of my bougainvillea plant. I remembered at that moment that I planted it close to my window on purpose, to remind me of Greece. I suddenly felt so happy and pleased with my life. I was doing for a living exactly what I always wanted to.

James and I kept talking for over half an hour. In the meantime, it got dark outside. We discussed the past lives he had revisited, and after that we talked about books again. When he left, I thought to myself how easy my job would be if every client was like him, wanting to know as much as the Universe can reveal. But then, every client is different and as my husband says *"it takes all sorts"*.

Integrity starts with loving yourself and being true to who you are, because you cannot possibly love dishonesty and fakeness. The Latin word *"integer"* says it all, *"being whole"* or *"being complete"*. In essence, aspiring to sincerity in life takes us on a road to high morals and to living a transparent life and ultimately to that inner peace we all search for.

Having a background in philosophy, when I refer to integrity as a system of moral values, I always point out the different approaches the American philosopher Ronald Dworkin and the British philosopher Herbert Lionel Adolphus Hart had on this subject. Whilst Dworkin argued that our own moral system – which we build our lives on - could be sometimes incorrect or even wrong, Hart believed that the main rule underlying any of our structure is based on the Rule of Recognition. In my view, the truth is somewhere in the middle. I believe that we build a personal system of ethics based on moral values passed on to us and agreed on initially. We add to it our own aspirations that start with real life examples or personal experiences. Then we continuously test the validity of morals based on their own efficacy. If the morals serve us to evolve, we accept them; if not, we look for others to replace them. It may be a sad perspective on ethical values, but it is as true as it gets nowadays when, in most cases, there is a thin line between black and white.

As I get older, integrity, with all it comprises - sincerity, loyalty, truth - is the value I aim most towards in the years I have left. If I can be that, I am complete indeed!

Karmic lesson 8

FUN

"You are allowed to be who you are"

Karly is one of my best friends. I first met her ten years ago when she contacted me for one of my services. I did my job well - as I usually do - and after that we kept in touch. We both lived in the biggest city in New Zealand and tried seeing each other from time to time. Then we both moved away to two smaller towns, over four hours apart. Despite the distance, our friendship grew and, a year later, I was overjoyed to find out that she planned moving to the city I had just recently moved to. In a short period of time, she found the perfect house a few minutes away from me. From then on, our friendship developed even more.

What I love about Karly is that she brings out the best in me... the very best in everybody she comes into contact with actually. With Karly, everything is simple. She is honest, understanding and nonjudgmental. Karly would never disappoint me and her friendship is one that I value more than any other relationship I have ever had.

In her late forties, she has that kind of beauty that would fit perfectly into the 1950s; beautiful curves, curly hair and a doll face with a heart shaped mouth. For me, she is a charismatic version of Marilyn Monroe... with darker hair. Bubbly, full of joy, Karly is always the life and soul of every party; her jokes are the funniest, her conversation the best, her laugh truly contagious.

If you believe that Karly is nothing other than fun, I have to argue that she is so much more than that. Very smart and professional, this bubble of joy was successfully teaching at one of the academies in Auckland. With her move to my city, she was in the process of deciding what she wanted to do in the years to follow. I knew she would succeed in whatever she wanted to do, because she was pleasant, smart, extremely skilled and an asset to the world.

I was thrilled when Karly approached me for a past life regression and booked her for a Friday at lunchtime. She had never had a regression before and I knew that this might cause her anxiety. Usually clients are excited when they make a booking and become anxious just before the session. Karly was no different, but a good chat between us brought out laughter and a relaxed state. I started inducing hypnosis and not in a million years would I have been prepared for what was to follow.

Karly: *"It's dark where I am. I am somewhere inside. I feel that I am in a cupboard."*

BC: *"How did you get in the cupboard?"*

Karly: *"It wasn't a game. I was hiding... I don't know why. I feel that I was in trouble."*

BC: *"Is it light enough in the cupboard to see your feet?"*

Kerry: *"Yes, my feet are smaller. I feel that they are child's feet."*

BC: *"Are you a boy or a girl?"*

Karly: *"I feel that I am a little boy."*

BC: *"How old you are?"*

Karly: *"Three years old."*

BC: *"Do you have any parents?"*

Karly: *"No. I feel that I am an orphan."*

BC: *"Are you in an orphanage?"*
Karly: *"Yes, in London."*
BC: *"Are there any children, orphans like you, who you recognize as being somebody in your present life?"*
Karly: *"Yes, there is a girl with blonde curly hair... a little girl. I know her. Feels like it's me too... yes, she is me too. I see her through a small hole in the wood. She is me too."*

Karly seemed surprised and I was wondering if the little boy and the girl with the blonde curly hair were twins. I suddenly remembered about the theory regarding the souls' division, but, to be perfectly honest, I had never experienced a regression in which a client remembered two parts of a soul that had reincarnated simultaneously. I therefore started asking myself if I was actually witnessing the proof of quantum entanglement. And whilst I kept wondering whether this was remarkable or just average, Karly seemed stuck in the moment. I realized that there was no other memory to be recalled from that lifetime, so I left it at that, but decided to come back to it later in the session.

BC: *"Let's leave this scene and move to a more relevant one as I count from three to one... three... two... and one... It's up to you what you want to remember, a memory from the same life or a totally different one."*

Before even responding, Karly became very serious. Her face was beautiful and denoted so much character. I loved this girl and realized how lucky I was to have her as a close friend.

Karly: *"I see an older woman. She looks older than she is... what she is wearing makes her look older... a tight corset... all black. I don't know why I remember her."*

BC: *"Perhaps it is important for you. Look at the surroundings. What do you see?"*

Karly: *"She is inside... in a house, standing in front of the front door. It's a really big house. I don't think that she is rich."*

BC: *"What is she doing in that house?"*

Karly: *"I think she is a teacher... quite rigid. They are no children around."*

BC: *"Is she married?"*

Karly: *"No. She is single. She has never been married."*

BC: *"So why is she in that house?"*

Karly: *"They know her. She works for these people."*

BC: *"So is she working with children?"*

Karly: *"Not anymore. I have the feeling that she now works in something related to funerals."*

There was something about that woman that frightened Karly. I couldn't really put my finger on what it might have been, but I knew that the very serious teacher may have played a role in one of her existences and I decided to find out what that was.

BC: *"Do you remember the country?"*

Karly: *"England... in London. Everything looks old."*

BC: *"Pick now another memory that may be relevant to you."*

Karly amazed me again. I expected her to continue sharing what she remembered about that rigid woman, but she jumped into another body in a totally different existence. Suddenly, she started smiling and giggling.

Karly: *"I am a lot happier now. I am young. I am twenty. I walk on the street. There is somebody who stops to see me. It's a man... he is cheeky. I don't know who he is."*

BC: *"That's fine. Keep walking."*

Karly: *"I wear a beautiful dress. It's summer."*

BC: *"If there is no other relevant memory, move in time to a scene that may be significant for you. It's up to you what you pick."*

Karly picked a scene back in time when she was younger. More proof that in the process of recalling memories in a past life, time doesn't necessarily follow a chronological, linear order.

Karly: *"I am five now. I am on the same street I walked when I was older."*

BC: *"Is there anybody with you?"*

Karly: *"No. I am by myself. I have a lollipop... it's big. Looks like a traditional lollipop... you know... white and red. I just got to my house. It's big. Wow... it's big. I live here... maybe work for these people..."*

BC: *"Do you know where this house may be?"*

Karly: *"I am in Savannah. Holy hell. I am black... a black girl."*

I listened to Karly and couldn't stop smiling. She had the most perfect skin I have ever seen in my whole life; her ivory skin looked like the finest porcelain. I just hoped that the little girl she had been in Savannah had the most amazing ebony skin.

BC: *"Are there any people around?"*

Karly: *"Many people. I recognize one of them. A girl."*

BC: *"Is she somebody in your present?"*

Karly: *"Yes, she is my sister now. She doesn't look like her now, but I know it's her. We are both picking cotton."*

BC: *"Are you happy?"*

Karly: *"Oh yes, very happy. Life is easy."*

BC: *"What is your name?"*

Karly: *"Isabelle."*

BC: *"Go now to the time when Isabelle is older."*

Karly: *"I am inside the house. I am a teenager. I am wearing black. I don't have any boy in my life... I don't have time. I see my sister outside."*

BC: *"If nothing happens, go now to another memory in the same lifetime as Isabelle."*

Karly: *"I am now in my own little house... a cottage. It's a little bit rundown, but I love it! I am sitting on a chair. I am so old!"*

BC: *"Do you have a male companion in your life?"*

Karly: *"No. I was too busy my whole life."*

BC: *"What happens next?"*

Karly: *"I am by myself. I am dying alone."*

BC: *"That's fine. Do you remember the lesson for the life you just revisited?"*

Karly: *"To bring people together with... fun!"*

As Karly was able to jump from one life to another, I made up my mind to continue the journey of her soul as long as time permitted. It was still early and I was able to spend more time with Karly. It was Friday anyway and my next client for that day was three hours away.

BC: *"Leave this life behind and revisit now another lifetime. Let me know when you are there."*

Karly: *"I am in the army, in the first line, where everything is happening. I am a boy. I am cheeky..."*

BC: *"How old are you?"*

Karly: *"Nineteen... in the first line...where it is all happening. Something happened to my leg."*

BC: *"Do you remember the year?"*

Karly: *"Yes... it's 1876. Belgium comes to my mind... I don't know why. I am Belgian. We are under fire."*

BC: *"What is your name?"*

Karly: *"Ian."*

BC: *"What do you see when you look around?"*

Karly: *"There are many of us there. There is a sergeant too."*

BC: *"Do you recognize any of these people as ones you know in the present?"*

Karly: *"The sergeant is my dad in the present."*

BC: *"So what happens?"*

Karly: *"He is yelling at us 'get out there!'. I am scared. My leg is hurting."*

I continued, ignoring Karly's concern about her leg, because deep down I knew that Ian might have been hurt in the battle.

BC: *"Do you have a girlfriend?"*

Karly: *"I have lots of girls. I am cheeky. I am fun!"*

BC: *"Tell me about the fight."*

Karly: *"We survive for now. It's quiet. I am in the front line and it catches me off guard. I am now down... I am out. I am floating."*

BC: *"Do you remember the lesson you had to learn in this life?"*

Karly: *"To have fun... fun... even in the worst times. Have fun! I respect the sergeant, but you don't have to be like him. Have fun! It was a short life, I was scared, but I had fun!"*

Before even guiding her to another lifetime, Karly surprised me again and jumped back into the body of the little boy hiding in a cupboard of an orphanage.

Karly: *"I am in the cupboard. They don't like me."*

BC: *"Why is that?"*

Karly: *"I am not good enough... they don't like me. My parents didn't want me either. I wasn't good enough for them either."*

BC: *"What do you remember about your parents?"*

Karly: *"They are not together anymore. I was a mistake. I was just not wanted."*

BC: *"What is the year?"*

Karly: *"1920. It feels like London. It's cold and foggy."*

BC: *"What happened to you?"*

Karly: *"I was in that cupboard for ages. I think I'm going to die in that cupboard... by myself. It started being scary; then I am just lying there. They don't like me...*

maybe because of my parents... I've come from sin. They like the girl with blonde curly hair."

Karly mentioned again the little girl she identified as herself too. I was more and more inclined to believe that they might have been twins in that reincarnation.

BC: *"That's fine. Do you remember what lesson may have been for this life?"*

Karly: *"I am enough. I am good. Have fun because you are good enough."*

BC: *"If there is nothing else to remember, see yourself now in another life."*

I just said the words and Karly pushed her chest out and started moving on the recliner. She was all smiles and she seemed happy. I had the feeling that I caught a sense of pride of the person she remembered she was in a past life.

Karly: *"I've been dancing. I am a Spanish dancer. I am stunning. I've got those castanets... Everyone is watching. I am Rosela. The place is full of music. I have dark skin. I am very self absorbed... very confidant."*

BC: *"Is there anybody around you who you recognize?"*

Karly: *"There are many faces I know, but not sure how. Wait! My friend Gina is here. She looks different but I feel that she is Gina. I know she is here."*

BC: *"Do you have any family?"*

Karly: *"I don't think so. I am strong by myself."*

BC: *"So you are dancing..."*

Karly: *"I am in the middle, dancing on the dance floor. I would be thirty... stunning! I made a fortune. I am pretty well off... my shoes are expensive. I have pretty good dancing shoes. Things are being paid for."*

BC: *"Is there any lover in your life?"*

Kerry: *"Oh yes."*

BC: *"Is he somebody in your present life?"*

Karly: *"Yes, he is my husband now... he is so familiar... But I had a few other lovers... many!"*

BC: *"Are you still dancing?"*

Karly: *"I am always dancing. I find it hard to stop because I love the attention. I am really beautiful... I am exotic."*

Karly suited her past incarnation as a dancer. She was as stunning as Rosela may have been.

BC: *"Move now to another scene when you may be a little bit older."*

Karly: *"Things are starting to ache. I am happy though. I am not dancing as much, but I can still do it."*

BC: *"Is your lover still around?"*

Karly: *"I believe that I got married. I feel that he doesn't seem to be around... but then I am older and I see a man bringing me tea. He is not the same lover... not the one who is my husband now. He is another man."*

BC: *"Can you recognize him?"*

Karly: *"Hmm... he is a guy I used to know from school, years ago."*

BC: *"So what happened to the one who is your husband now?"*

Karly: *"I think he left me. I feel like he did. I was too much..."*

BC: *"Any children?"*

Karly: *"No, I couldn't... I danced..."*

BC: *"Revisit now the very last moments just before your death."*

Karly: *"I am just sitting there... just passing away in my sleep... peacefully..."*

BC: *"What was your lesson for this lifetime?"*

Karly: *"Do what you want to do... have the attention... embrace life... you are sexy and gorgeous... you are allowed to be who you are... it's all about fun. Have fun!"*

Karly's regression was coming to an end. I wasn't ready to stop it though because I badly wanted to know why she remembered memories about that rigid teacher. I supposed that there was a connection between that woman and one of the bodies Karly's soul incarnated into. I knew I had to know the truth and I was sure that this was important for Karly too.

BC: *"Now I want you to go back to that lifetime as a girl with curly hair and the teacher, wearing the corset. Revisit that lifetime now."*

Karly: *"She is an angry person."*

BC: *"Why do you think she is angry?"*

Karly: *"Oh dear, I see an old boyfriend... I knew him in that lifetime too. I feel that he wasn't honest to that teacher. She is hurt and she doesn't trust anybody... She doesn't like anybody..."*

BC: *"Is that woman you?"*

Karly: *"No! I am that girl with the blonde curly hair!"*

BC: *"So who is she?"*

Karly: *"She is my mother now. She is so mean! So mean! She was part of my life then. I am the little girl with the curly hair... the orphan."*

BC: *"That's fine. What happens to that mean woman?"*

Karly: *"She slips over and she cannot get up. She is by herself... and she dies. There is water... she dies in such a weird way... drowning in a little bit of water. Her clothes are so heavy and she cannot... life is just so weird... it's dark, like in a tunnel. Her shoe is slippery and when she falls, she hits the ground very hard."*

BC: *"Look back to your life. Is there anybody who you recognize?"*

Karly: *"I know her. She is my mother in my current life. I feel that woman was a teacher at the orphanage. She didn't like me and she didn't like the little boy who died in the cupboard. She was so mean."*

BC: *"So what happens to you after this woman dies?"*

Karly: *"I am finally happy. I am wanted. I am happier... so happy and free. I am still in the orphanage and they like me and I have a good life."*

Most of the time, I learn more from my clients than they would from me. They may not realize that though. Karly reminded me that life is short indeed and fun should be a part of it. It may not be random that she remembered lives in which fun was primordial even to survive. However, not in my wildest dreams, would I have thought that fun could be a lesson rather than a blessing, but again Karly proved me wrong... and for that and many other reasons, I am forever grateful to her!

These days, everything seems to be about fun. The Internet is full of it and even social media is build around it. We believe that we need fun in our jobs and in our personal lives and often confuse fun with joy and enjoyment. Fun, however, brings a level of playfulness that indicates taking life easy. For me, fun means living in the moment, in a state of perfect gratification, and letting the future unfold naturally.

We believe that we need people to entertain us, and forget that we can enjoy ourselves by doing what we most love doing. It is not the job that needs to amuse us; it is us who have to get pleasure from doing it. If that cannot happen, we will live a life of misery, being continuously bored and unhappy.

Fun, in my opinion does not relate to superficiality or mediocrity. There is a level of vital seriousness to fun as well. Embracing every breath in and out with excitement and being grateful for what this is, means living in a state of fun. Because at the end of the day, you cannot inhale the past and definitely cannot exhale the future.

Karmic lesson 9

PROSPERITY

"Build an empire"

George definitely suits his manly old-fashioned name. He arrived for the appointment - booked a month in advance - wearing a very stylish and traditional navy blue three-piece suit and a perfectly ironed cream shirt. His posture oozed confidence and a certain financial achievement. He filled in the forms refusing my pen. Instead he took out a very fancy pen from one of his suit pockets.

As it was a very hot day, I asked him if he would feel more comfortable without the jacket and waistcoat, but he looked straight into my eyes and said that he was used to wearing a suit every day, so I left it at that. Then he told me about his very successful business and his busy schedule.

As he talked, I wondered what made this forty-three year old man - who looked like he was on top of the world - book a past life regression. After more than ten minutes, I still hadn't got to the point of understanding why he was in my practice, because he talked about his professional achievements, money, a few central properties he owned, the very engaging social life he had and physical health to be envied. On top of it all, he was an extremely attractive and well-presented man. *"I don't have anybody to share all this with"*, he admitted and for the first time he dropped the mask of success, one that I guessed he wore every day... day in, day out.

George then talked about all the romantic relationships he had ever had; all of the women he had dated so far enjoyed the lifestyle he was able to offer them, rather than wanting him for who he was. He said that he respected and was loyal to all the women who entered into his life, but he felt that nothing worked because none of them stuck around for too long. I looked at him and thought to myself that there may have been a hidden side to him, or perhaps his past lovers were all blind. *"You are my last resort of finding out why and turning my luck around"*, George said.

George wasn't an easy subject to bring into trance and I knew that he resisted just because he was used to being in control; but everybody can be hypnotized and he was no different. After a good half an hour, George began sharing memories from a life he remembered nothing about prior to the regression.

George: *"I am a young woman... maybe sixteen. I have long curly black hair and light colored eyes... not blue... not green... more like gold color. A very beautiful girl! My skin is very pale because I don't like staying too long in the sun; I look after my skin."*

BC: *"What are you wearing?"*

George: *"A long creamy color dress with a black bow at the back. The dress is very pretty... but cheap!"*

BC: *"What do you mean by that?"*

George: *"I am quite poor, but that I have to change."*

BC: *"In what way?"*

George: *"I am very ambitious and I want to be rich. I am going to New York and, when I get there, I will make money... loads of it!"*

BC: *"Are you on the way to New York?"*

George: *"Yes. I am on a boat... almost there... two or perhaps three hours away."*

BC: *"Are you traveling with family?"*

George: *"No. My parents are back in Italy. I ran away. They wanted me to marry a man whose family they knew... he is a good man, but he is not rich and I want to be! So I met this man who had two tickets, one for him and one for his fiancé. I ran away with him."*

BC: *"How come you are traveling with him instead of his fiancé?"*

George: *"She is my cousin Elena. Our mothers are sisters, but so different. Her mother is kind; mine is very strict. Elena had to marry him and then emigrate to America, but changed her mind. She didn't want to leave her family behind. She was afraid of going away with him, I guess. I wasn't. I met him and asked him if I could have the other ticket. He said yes so I ran away with him."*

BC: *"Can you recognize Elena or her fiancé as being somebody you know in the preset life?"*

George: *"Elena is one of my girlfriends... we stopped talking a long time ago. The man is another girlfriend of mine. In my present life, I proposed to them both, but they rejected me. They thought that I wasn't ready for marriage."*

As I listened to George, I realized that I had never had such a chatty client like him; at least not during a past life regression. George was so coherent and willing to explain everything he remembered, and this side to him was more appealing than who he actually was now.

BC: *"So tell me more about the man you are traveling with."*

George: *"His name is David. He is a good man; hard worker, soft... good man. He wants to start a restaurant in America. He is a good cook. He wants to teach me to cook and work for him."*

BC: *"Do you love him?"*

George: *"Not that way. He is like a brother to me. He feels the same way. We are not in a romantic relationship."*

BC: *"What is your name?"*

George: *"Daniela. They named me after my grandmother on my father's side. She was ambitious like me. She wanted to live somewhere else, but then she got pregnant and had to marry my grandfather. She wasn't happy."*

BC: *"Is she somebody you know in the current life?"*

George: *"Yes. She is my mother."*

BC: *"Tell me about the other passengers."*

George: *"There are many people... all poor... all searching for a better life. We travelled for weeks. Some children died and it was so sad seeing their parents cry. I made a friend; her name is Laura and she is from a village next to mine. She is nineteen and knows somebody in a big city in America. She hopes she can stay there for a while."*

BC: *"Do you recognize her?"*

George: *"She is a woman I had a blind date with, organized by my best friend."*

I guided George to that moment when Daniela arrived in New York and his face lit up.

George: *"It is so different to the way I thought it might be. We are on the other side now. I don't understand the language."*

Then George moved automatically to another memory. He looked happy, so different to the way he had been when he walked in my practice.

George: *"We have a small room... just a bed and an old table. David got a job in a small restaurant. They like him there. He introduced me to his boss and I now clean the restaurant and wash dishes. We are saving every penny."*

BC: *"What are you saving your money for?"*

George: *"We want our own restaurant. I learnt to cook, but David is much better. We can make it together."*

BC: *"What is the year?"*

George: *"I think it's 1806. The place is called Manhattan."*

A few minutes later, George jumped five years in time.

George: *"I am twenty-one now. Our boss got really sick and then died and we inherited the restaurant. He had no family. Just before he died, he talked to us about the restaurant and he gave us some money too. We have a business and money now. We saved a lot and we inherited a lot. We don't live in that small room anymore. I live in a room at the back of the restaurant, so we are saving even more money. David met somebody. They want to get married."*

BC: *"Who is she?"*

George: *"She is Laura, the girl I met on the boat. We came across her again a year after we arrived. Her friend didn't help her out, so I did. Then, when we inherited the restaurant, we gave her a job. She is a very loyal girl and I love her like a sister. I am happy for David and her."*

George made my work easier than any other client I have ever had. He answered my questions with the kind of detail I've never experienced before in my career.

BC: *"And you? Did you meet anybody?"*

George: *"No. I don't want that. I want a career. Not many women own a business. I do!"*

BC: *"Do you keep in touch with your parents?"*

George: *"I wrote them two letters. They never responded. They cannot write anyway. The schoolteacher would have to write them, but I don't think they wanted to keep in touch with me. I sent them some money too, through somebody who went back to Italy. That would help them survive for a while. They might feel embarrassed I ran away."

BC: *"As I count from one to three, I want you to move to another memory."*

I looked at George whilst I was counting. He seemed so comfortable with the life he revisited and, to some degree, it actually felt like his present life. He wanted success and abundance first. For me the only difference was that in his current life he searched for a partner, but I wasn't totally convinced that he was putting his whole heart into the process of finding a soul mate. Maybe he wanted to create rules in a relationship in the same manner as he did within his business, or perhaps he was just unlucky.

George: *"I am twenty-nine now and very beautiful. I wear my long black hair down. I have taste and I pick stunning dresses and pieces of jewelry... I have money to afford them all. I don't have champagne taste on a beer budget! There are a few men who proposed to me, but I am not sure I want to get married. I still live in the little room at the back of the restaurant and am saving all my money. I am very good with money."*

BC: *"What about David?"*

George's voice broke down as he answered my question and I realized that he was just about to share a sad memory.

George: *"David died last year. He got suddenly sick, poor guy. Life was good for him. He moved to a house with a garden and planned having children. Laura and he were very in love, but then he died. I couldn't mourn for very long, as I had to keep the business going and help Laura get through. She now owns their house, but I pay for all the expenses."*

BC: *"Tell me about the restaurant."*

George: *"Business is good. I expanded and have more tables in the restaurant. Everything is spotless and the food is good. I opened a bakery next to the restaurant and people travel long distances to buy from me. I have five people working for me. I cook and supervise everybody and late at night, just before I fall asleep, I dream of expanding my business even more."

BC: *"In what way?"*

George: *"I want a flower shop next to the bakery and I've already got the space. Somebody is painting the walls there and renovating. Then there is that young girl who will sell flowers for me."*

BC: *"Do you recognize her?"*

George: *"Yes, another of my former girlfriends now."*

Without instructing him, George moved to another moment in the lifetime as Daniela. He seemed excited to share good news with me, so I let him talk without interrupting.

George: *"I do even better than planned. I am still young... thirty-two. I own almost the whole street. I have shop after shop... all sorts... restaurants, bakery, flower shop, vegetable shop, fashion shop... all sorts. Women don't make it this far in business. I did! Some men want me gone, but it's too late now. I have power! Alessandro is here too."*

BC: *"Alessandro?"*

George: *"Alessandro is the man I had to marry back in Italy. He left for America around the same time I did. He said that nothing kept him back home. I met him again in America last summer. I didn't know he was in New York. He has a construction company and is doing very well... many people working for him. He proposed today. I said yes."*

BC: *"Do you love him?"*

George: *"Very much. It's not a teenage love. I know what I want and he knows too. We are better off together.*

We built good businesses and we may go bigger together. He built a house and I will be moving in with him."

BC: *"Are you happy?"*

George: *"Very much so. Excited. We are alike. We think the same."*

BC: *"I want you to move now to another memory in the same life and, when you are there, tell me what you see, hear or feel."*

George: *"I am older now... not older than forty though. I have a son. I called him David, in the memory of my friend. He has curly black hair and dark eyes. He is maybe five or six. We live in a nice house built by Alessandro. There is a swing in the middle of the garden."*

BC: *"How is the business going?"*

George: *"Great. Many shops, very busy."*

BC: *"How is Alessandro?"*

George: *"He has been back to Italy and took some money to my parents. They are old and fragile and we help them out. I haven't seen them since I left. Maybe I will one day, but I am very busy and who knows..."*

BC: *"Who knows... I want you now to move to the moment of your death."*

George: *"I am very old... eighty-three. My joints are full of arthritis. I worked too hard... but I accomplished everything I dreamed of. I am in my own bed. David is here with me... and his wife."*

BC: *"And Alessandro?"*

George: *"He died two years ago. He was a good man. We worked well together. We were business partners and very good friends. We respected each other. I ran away from him and I got together with him. You cannot run away from what's meant to be."*

BC: *"Take your time now and experience your death."*

George kept quiet for a few minutes before he started talking again.

George: *"I am above my body now. I hear voices and see a bright light. There is so much love here. There are no people around. I don't know how to describe what I see. There are entities... light entities. They don't speak, but I understand what they say. They are pleased with how I lived. I was fair and helped people. I learnt everything I was supposed to."*

BC: *"Do you remember what your lesson was for the lifetime you revisited?"*

George: *"I had to learn about prosperity... abundance. I learnt to build an empire. I did well and I had a great life."*

The sun was going down as I finished the session and the whole room was filled with an enigmatic red light. It was nice and comfortable inside whilst outside the temperature was still very high. I heard the birds making weird noises and thought to myself that, if we were lucky, it may rain overnight.

I turned to George and asked him about the feelings his regression may have brought forward. He looked confused and took his time before answering. I knew that the issue that brings a client into my practice may not be sorted right after a regression, but there may be clarity in identifying the problem itself. This was spot on in George's case. He thought that the lifetime he revisited brought light to the mystery in his present life. He admitted feeling that the energy he sent out to the women he used to date might have blocked the possibility of them accepting to settle down with him. *"Maybe they thought I was married to my work and I couldn't fit them into my busy schedule",* he admitted. *"Or perhaps you proposed to the wrong women",* I answered.

George left my practice in a rather happy mood and I didn't hear back from him for a while. I emailed at some stage, but had no reply. Then, one day, a few months later, George rang. He met 'the one' he said, and to be perfectly honest, I was thrilled for him. He talked about her for a while, then said that his new love is a woman he met a long time ago on a blind date organized by one of his friends. They met by accident years after their first date and fell in love. I so wanted to ask him if she was a reincarnation of Alessandro... but I didn't.

When we refer to prosperity, money and assets come first to our minds. Abundance, however, is much more than that. I personally believe that abundance is a mindset and that we attract what our own minds see. We become prosperous if we decide to receive abundance in every aspect of our lives. You've probably heard about the Law of Abundance, which states that bounty is unlimited and in order to receive ampleness in relationships, career or finance you need to attract it by manifesting your wishes, making the right choices and acting upon them. In other words, you reap what you sow.

You've perhaps also heard about the Law of Attraction, mostly referred to as the Law of New Thought. It became more popular with the 2006 release of Rhonda Bryne's book *"The Secret"*, which was based on the idea that we attract what we emit; therefore positive thoughts attract profitability and even opulence. The topic was, however, used for the first time in the nineteen century by Phineas Quimby, an American spiritual teacher, who developed the theory behind the New Thought. He believed that the mind is stronger than the body and can even heal physical unaligned issues. Quimby proved his method by testing it on himself early in life when he was diagnosed with tuberculosis and successfully treated himself by using the power of his mind.

For me, the strongest example of attracting health in abundance is Milton Erickson, an American psychologist and psychiatrist, considered the most revolutionary figure in hypnotherapy. Even pronouncing his name excites me, as I am a follower of the Ericksonian techniques in hypnotherapy and am a huge admirer of his work. Erickson healed himself early in his life, at the age of seventeen, when he was diagnosed with polio, by using his brain in remembering body/muscular memories.

There is no doubt that our brains can be reprogrammed to visualize - and therefore attract - positivity in every aspect of our lives. However, we so often see people who struggle, and in many cases it is not their fault; but sometimes it is. Not everybody is unfortunate; some people got to where they are now because of poor choices, whether associating themselves with people who are not right for them or mimicking other fellows' failures. Abundance comes in many forms and attracting it starts with changing our mindsets, or even powering up our brains for success.

BRIGITTE CALLOWAY

Karmic lesson 10

DUTY

"Love should overstep duty"

Cora is a stunning woman. In her early thirties, she could turn every head on the street. Tall, with long legs and a very small waist, Cora is a stunner! When I first met her, I thought that every man would do anything to have her... but after breaking up from a long-term relationship, Cora remained single and no man was rushing to secure a place in her life. I wasn't sure her explanation that she only wanted to focus on raising her three children was the whole truth. Because she wanted to be perceived as being comfortable with her life, I rather believed that she might have been scared of learning and accommodating any new habits of an upcoming potential partner.

The conversation with Cora flowed naturally and, in the half an hour before the regression, she told me more about her life. She spoke about her spirituality and her beliefs in such an organic manner that would have embarrassed others. Then Cora moved on to discuss her fear of not being in control. She believed that giving in to life itself would take her to a position where she would be less in charge of her destiny.

I usually find that our stubbornness in controlling our life paths and fate, makes us more confused about our meaning. Cora, on the other hand, believed that whilst in control, nothing bad could happen to her and her children. However, she was more afraid of the positives than the negatives. *"I have that fear of not being able to control the good side"*, she said at some stage; then she elaborated on the causes of her panic, but everything I heard demonstrated her determination to try this and that and, if nothing worked, try something else again. In the search of her inner peace, Cora tried everything and each of her experiences created even more questions for her about how to achieve the calm and tranquility of mind she desperately searched for. Her fear, or maybe anxiety, was accentuated as a result and she found herself back to square one after each new experience.

As she talked about her daily life - as well as entities and spirits she believed she encountered in her meditation and in other spiritual practices - I wondered if the cause of her restless search was the fear that bad things have their roots in good ones. So after our chat, I asked her to find a comfortable position on the recliner and the whole hypnotic regression started.

Cora: *"I see a big house with dark walls. As I go inside, I see that the wall paper is green with some brown patterns."*

BC: *"I want you to look down to you feet and notice if they are smaller or larger."*

Cora: *"They are smaller... feet of a little girl with red shoes on."*

BC: *"What are you wearing?"*

Cora: *"A dress, check pattern dress. The fabric is not soft at all."*

BC: *"What else can you tell me about you?"*

Cora: *"I have dark brown hair with gold highlights... just passing my shoulders. I have brown eyes. I am a five year old girl."*

BC: *"Do you remember your name?"*

Cora: *"It starts with an M."*

BC: *"Don't worry if you cannot remember it. Who else is with you in the house?"*

Cora: *"My mom and dad are here somewhere, but I don't see them at the moment."*

BC: *"Do you know where your house is?"*

Cora: *"It's outside of a city... a big city."*

I suddenly realized that Cora was expressing herself as a five year old girl and that there was no way for her to remember her exact location. Therefore I decided to ask her more details later in the session.

BC: *"Tell me about your room in the house."*

Cora: *"I see a large window and some children's books. There are toys too... and a bed."*

Suddenly Cora moved to a totally different time in that life.

Cora: *"I am twenty-three now. I am in a dining room... attending a party. I am wearing a green satin dress with long sleeves and creamy satin leggings."*

BC: *"Do you remember the year?"*

Cora: *"Early 1920s."*

BC: *"Do you have a boyfriend?"*

Cora: *"There is a boy playing the piano. I am sitting behind him. He is my boyfriend."*

BC: *"Can you recall his name?"*

Cora: *"John."*

BC: *"What about your name; can you remember it now?"*

Cora: *"Martha."*

BC: *"Tell me more about yourself."*

Cora: *"I study Literature... I have a great future ahead. I don't work and still live with my parents. My mother needs my help..."*

BC: *"Tell me about the party."*

Cora: *"I am smoking in the room. There are many youngsters, drinking and smoking. It's fun!"*

BC: *"Move now to another scene in the same lifetime as Martha. You can pick any memory you wish."*

Cora: *"I am nursing my mother. I am in my late thirties... maybe thirty-nine... still living in the same house."*

BC: *"What is wrong with your mother?"*

Cora: *"She is coughing... there is something wrong with her lungs."*

BC: *"Is she somebody you know in the present life?"*

Cora: *"She is my mom now."*

BC: *"Is your father still around?"*

Cora: *"He is always away on business. I don't see him much."*

BC: *"What about that guy John?"*

Cora: *"He thought I was too good for him. He moved on. I've heard that he is happy now... he wasn't when we broke up."*

BC: *"Do you recognize him as being somebody you know now?"*

Cora: *"He looks very familiar... hmm... very familiar."*

BC: *"Is there any other man in your life?"*

Cora: *"No. I never really left home. I wasn't as confident as I should have been. I was still dependent on my parents. My mother needed me around."*

BC: *"Move now to another scene in the same life and tell me what you remember."*

Cora: *"I am in mom's bedroom. My mother is freezing cold. She was very sick... she is dead now."*

BC: *"Have you made any promise to your mother before she died?"*

Cora: *"Yes... to always do the right thing... no matter what."*

BC: *"Move now to a memory just a few days after your mother died."*

Cora: *"My dad wants to sell the house. He is not coming back. So I don't know where to go. My father has already got somebody else in his life... another woman."*

Cora kept silent for a few seconds, then started talking again. I looked at her and noticed that the stunning woman she was suddenly looked so tired and hopeless. I understood that her memories were sad.

Cora: *"Yes, the house is gone now. I am in an apartment in the old part of a city... in Poland. I am not very happy... it's all because of my father."*

BC: *"Do you recognize him as being somebody in the present life?"*

Cora: *"He is my ex husband now."*

BC: *"What about his new partner?"*

Cora: *"Yes, she is my sister now."*

BC: *"How do you survive?"*

Cora: *"I work in a kind of cafe... it is definitely not easy though..."*

BC: *"Do you have anybody in your life?"*

Cora: *"No. I am very bitter now... grumpy. I could have had a great future...my life was supposed to be great. I have to work hard instead. I am not happy at all. I am alone."*

BC: *"How old are you now?"*

Cora: *"Fifty-six."*

BC: *"Did you ever see your father after your mom passed away?"*

Cora: *"No. He didn't want any contact with me. He had other children."*

BC: *"Go now to the very last moments in that life, without experiencing any stress."*

Cora: *"I am in hospital. I have a lung problem... like my mother did. I am very old. My skin is all scabby and bruised. I can't breathe properly."*

BC: *"Look back at your life now. How was it?"*

Cora: *"Not happy! It was a very sad life... very sad, not accomplished."*

BC: *"Experience now your soul leaving your body and, as you do that, I want you to remember if there is any residual energy you are carrying into the present."*

Cora: *"There is a letter that I wrote to John."*

BC: *"What did you write in that letter?"*

Cora: *"I promised that I would come to him and marry him. My father found out about it, so I couldn't go. I couldn't keep my promise, but I wonder how my life would have been with him."*

BC: *"Try to remember again if you recognize John as somebody present in your current life."*

Cora: *"Oh yes. He is my ex boyfriend."*

BC: *"Do you remember the lesson you had to learn as Martha?"*

Cora: *"Duty.... love should be stronger than duty... love should overstep duty."*

For some people, living a life for others may seem like a sacrifice, but Cora understood why she dedicated a whole past existence to her mother. She said that her present was pretty similar because she only focused on her children, forgetting or perhaps ignoring her own needs. A new partner was therefore impossible to fit into a structured life where things had a certain order and where Cora was in charge.

Cora and I moved the conversation around children and we shared our experiences as mothers. As much as I want to, it is not my place as a hypnotherapist to give life advice to my clients. I am there for them during the whole therapy process; if it's a traditional hypnotherapy one or a past life regression hypnosis, but I don't feel that I can say that my experience should be my clients' ones too. We are all different. However, I clicked with Cora and understood that motherhood could sometimes, if not always, overshadow every other aspect in a woman's life.

I never heard from Cora after the regression. I saw her once whilst driving in the city, but couldn't stop the car to talk to her. I noticed, however, that she looked very well presented and quite rested, and hoped for a second that she was going out for a catch up with her friends or a mysterious date. Who knows?

Duty doesn't necessarily mean that we are obliged to do certain things; it may also refer to the level of responsibility or commitment we have in different moments in our lives. We are responsible for our own actions and destiny, not for other people's actions. We don't have to do anything against our own beliefs and we don't need to do anything against other peoples' credence. In my opinion, the only duty we have is towards preserving and saving lives.

We feel that we have to fit in, no matter where in the world we live, whether at work or in our social groups. We don't really. We feel obliged to credit people and be accepted. Nobody asks us to be accountable for things that don't belong to us, or that we cannot control. Duty is a value; therefore related to an ethical system. There is no real duty outside what is morally expected from us.

As per its origin in Latin, *"debitum"*, duty refers to an assumption to do something. This expectation can *"destroy a man more quickly"*, said Friedrich Nietzsche, the German philosopher, who was against everything that comes out of duty. On the contrary, the Roman philosopher Cicero believed that duty could be an effect of our own expectations in regards to what we believe we are supposed to do.

The concept of duty is different in various cultures. If in feudal Japan, a samurai was proud to sacrifice himself in the name of duty and honor; an arranged marriage in other cultures may be seen as a humble acceptance of the way life is supposed to follow its flow, as well as a mandatory task to keep this life's course intact.

We live in societies where rules are already set in place and we feel obliged, even honored, to follow them. It is only right to do so in the aim of love, tolerance, empathy and compassion, and it is fair to follow morals that conserve life because at the end of the day nothing is more important than life itself.

Karmic lesson 11

KINDNESS

"Living for others"

October falls mid spring in New Zealand, a time of the year when the shades of green are infinite. Last year though, it rained for many days in a row and it seemed like winter. For me, born in a country with four seasons, the only difference between winter and the other seasons in Aotearoa is the amount of rain and maybe a few degrees Celsius up or down.

It was in October last year when I met Natalie. When she booked her appointment, Natalie said that she couldn't seem to stay focused on what she wanted and that she strongly believed that a past life regression would help her discover why. She arrived wearing a beautiful Titian red colored dress, and the quality of the fabric revealed that she had class, rather than the fact that she was able to afford expensive things. She was a well-presented woman, one who knew who she was and what she wanted from life.

In her early forties, Natalie was wiser than her age suggested. She seemed to have experienced loads in her life and had a special way of understanding everything and everybody. When I met her, she owned an alternative medical business and was very accepting about healing through natural and holistic therapies. However, she may have lost focus somewhere on the way and wondered what her next step was. She badly wanted to rekindle her passion, either by doing what she always did or finding excitement in something else. I admire people who want to make a change in the world and Natalie was one of them. She was logical, practical and very down to earth.

While I started conducting her to a relaxed stage, the sky opened up and it was pouring down. The rain outside was noisy and I was concerned that this might distract Natalie, but she didn't seem to care.

Natalie: *"I see horses... strong horses."*
BC: *"How many horses do you see?"*
Natalie: *"Five... they are white and dirty."*
BC: *"Can you see your feet?"*
Natalie: *"Yes. I have smaller feet. I am barefoot. I wear a skirt, maybe brownish color."*
BC: *"Is there anything around that catches your attention?"*
Natalie: *"I see stone walls... and stables. It looks like a stone courtyard. I know there is a house too, but cannot see it clearly. There are people working around me. I don't feel that I know them."*
BC: *"Do you know where this property may be?"*
Natalie: *"In Scotland."*
BC: *"So you're in Scotland. What is your name?"*
Natalie: *"Bridget... I am Bridget."*
BC: *"What can you recall about yourself as Bridget?"*
Natalie: *"I am ten years old. I remember having a father. He is a big man. My mother is gone... She died."*
BC: *"Do you have any siblings?"*
Natalie: *"I have an older brother. His name is Michael."*

BC: *"Just focus on your brother for a moment. Is he anybody you know in the present?"*

Natalie: *"Oh, he is my son."*

BC: *"Your son... Leave this memory now and move to another relevant one in the same life as Bridget. How old are you now?"*

Natalie: *"I am in my twenties. My hair is red and long and I have blue eyes."*

BC: *"Do you have a boyfriend, a fiancé or husband?"*

Natalie: *"No. I am single."*

BC: *"What about your brother Michael. Is he married?"*

Natalie: *"He is single too."*

BC: *"Tell me what you see, hear or feel now."*

Natalie: *"I am in the kitchen. I am cooking for my family... for my father and my brother... happy life..."*

BC: *"I will take you now to a scene in the same lifetime when you may be older, as I count from one to three. How old are you now?"*

Whilst I was counting, the rain continued to pour down. The noise outside was very loud, but Natalie still didn't seem to care.

Natalie: *"Not much older... still in my twenties... just a few years older. Still single... still in the kitchen... still cooking for my family. I am wearing a white shirt."*

BC: *"Can you recall what year it is?"*

Natalie: *"Yes. It's 1780."*

BC: *"Look around now. Do you live in a small or a big house?"*

Natalie: *"Just a cottage... but we have enough here."*

I waited for a few minutes, but Natalie didn't seem prepared to share more details about her home in the 1780s, so I asked her to move somewhere later in time. She started talking immediately.

Natalie: *"I am outside picking something... picking greens. There is nobody around. My brother is at the stables. Maybe my father is not around anymore because I don't sense him at all."*

BC: *"Is it a happy or a sad life?"*

Natalie: *"Happy... hmm... and lonely life. "*

BC: *"That's fine. I want you to find yourself in the very last moments of your life as Bridget. How old are you?"*

Nicky: *"Old... very old. I am in the cottage preparing some medicine. I am alone. There is nobody around. It's getting dark. Then I go inside and lie down on my bed."*

BC: *"Go on..."*

Natalie: *"I just go to sleep... and don't wake up. I die of old age."*

BC: *"That's fine. Let your soul float above your body and, whilst you float, I want you to tell me everything that happens."*

Natalie: *"I see sand. I don't hear voices, but I feel things."*

BC: *"What exactly do you feel?"*

Natalie: *"I feel love... love!"*

BC: *"Do you feel any messages in regards to the lesson you had to learn in that lifetime?"*

Natalie: *"Yes... kindness... living for others. I learnt to be kind with my family."*

BC: *"Did you accomplish that task?"*

Natalie: *"Yes. They tell me I did."*

BC: *"Who are they?"*

Natalie: *"Angels maybe."*

BC: *"Is there any contract or promise you feel you may have made as Bridget, that you carried in the present?"*

Natalie: *"Yes. I promised to look after Michael. This is all I've done my whole life."*

When a session finishes, I sometimes wonder how my clients can so naturally understand the life they have revisited. For Natalie too, everything seemed crystal clear. We chatted for a while whilst the noise made by the rain got even louder. Out the window, everything looked gray; just one of those days that never ends. Natalie talked about the memories she recalled and her eyes were so shiny. I understood instantly that the spark was what made her even more interesting. She was a fascinating young woman in search of her own destiny. If only she knew how smart and different she was.

Natalie made me think about the contrast between what we wish to do in this life and what we actually do. The two shouldn't be based on circumstances and opportunities which life throws our way. There is always a way out. There is always a chance that could take us to where we want to be. Life itself is built on options and choices rather than on occasions. Life is full of opportunities we could grab.

We haven't kept in touch; it would have been difficult anyway because Natalie lived quite far from me. However, I often ask myself if she changed her career, or made her practice a focus, because for me Natalie's reason for going through a regression was finding answers with regards to her job. But whatever she may have chosen to do since the regression, I was sure she would have achieved it, because Natalie was exactly that: a smart woman who knew herself and her limitless potential.

When I consider kindness, my mother always comes to my mind. There was a deep level of generosity in her that, combined with her natural gentleness, made her the most affectionate person I have ever met. She was even kind when she punished me for stupid things I may have done. She set an example of warmth, care and understanding. It was never hard for her to be kind; for the loving and compassionate person she was, it just came naturally.

In most cases, we associate kindness with tenderness, gentleness and softness, omitting that we may not be born with any of these qualities. We learn to have benignity and we definitely need practice to become kind. A kind person is not one who puts their head down whilst swallowing every evil that may come from other people; a kind person is compassionate, friendly and generous, whilst always acting on love. But most of all, a kind human has a warmth that can change people. My mother was just that.

Some people believe that kindness is a moral value and they may be right. Like them, the Chinese philosopher Confucius considered kindness to be one of the five main values one can possess alongside gravity, generosity, sincerity and earnestness. His humanistic teachings were focused on self-development virtues and ethical behavior. Same values were taken over by Ruism or Confucianism, which is a way of thinking focused on the concept of unity between divine and self.

I however believe that kindness is a product of our own behavior and, as much as we experience compassion, empathy and love, we have to change ourselves to adopt this virtue. I don't base my opinion on anything other than my personal experiences, and again, on the brightness my mother surrounded herself with.

Karmic lesson 12
HOPE

"Hope keeps us alive"

I met Fay more than a year ago, very soon after I moved to this city. I liked her then and I like her now. In her late thirties, Fay is a soft and delicate person. Her pale complexion and very thin body brings back memories from my childhood. Back then, I had a book I loved dearly, which featured illustrations about creatures who were half women-half angels. Fay is angelic indeed.

Fay is a holistic therapist and a good friend. We don't see each other often and, when we do, we don't share very intimate aspects of our lives. However, I know that she cares about me and she is concerned about the whole wide world. Empathy is probably her strength. Fay's partner is one of the subjects I presented in my first book *"You have lived many times"*, a guy who become a friend after being a client... or the other way around. I first regressed Fay last year and never thought that she would ask for more. But she did!

I mostly keep in touch with Fay on one of the social media channels and one Saturday morning I wasn't surprised to get a message from her, but I was almost dazed when I read it. She asked for another past life regression explaining that she may have reached crossroads. She felt blocked in any decision she wanted to take and confused about her whole life in general. I didn't hesitate to book her in for the next available appointment I was able to offer.

She came in wearing a long summery creamy-yellow dress that made her look even more fragile. Her partner was with her and I felt that she needed support and somebody to lean on. She explained that her troubled last few months started with her father having a stroke and I understood that she was very close to her father. Then she talked about not finding her way in life and even about not seeing the light at the end of the tunnel. She also referred to the fact that she felt her body aching without any reasons, which was quite unusual for a person like her because, even if she looked fragile and delicate, Fay was a fighter and a strong woman.

I kept the whole process of inducing trance simple because I'd already hypnotized Fay in the past and I knew that she was an easy subject. A few minutes later, she started sharing memories from one of her soul's past lives.

Fay: *"My feet are so heavy... there may be something wrong with them. I feel that they are smaller. I may be a little girl. I wear a blue dress. I have blue eyes and blonde hair. My skin is very pale."*

BC: *"How old are you?"*

Fay: *"I am nine years old."*

BC: *"Where are you now?"*

Fay: *"I am standing on the floor. There is nobody around. I don't think that I want to be there. It's not very comfortable."*

BC: *"Do you know why?"*

Fay: *"No. I just know that I don't want to be there."*

BC: *"What can you recall about your family?"*

Fay: *"I don't see any of my parents. I have an older sister. She is not around either."*

BC: *"What is your name?"*

Fay: *"Esme is my name."*

BC: *"I want you to move now to another experience in that lifetime. Tell me what you remember when you are there."*

I thought that Fay would remember something about Esme being older, but she went back in time to a scene when she was younger.

Fay: *"I am in a bed.... My legs are heavy! I may be five now. It's night."*

BC: *"Tell me about the room."*

Fay: *"It's pretty. The walls are white and the bed coverings have flower patterns."*

BC: *"Are your parents around?"*

Fay: *"I don't know where my parents are. They are never around. I know that they are alive. They may have left me in my grandmother's care. She is lovely. I remember now... yes, my parents left."*

BC: *"Do you recognize your grandmother as being somebody you know in the present?"*

Fay: *"Yes, she is my dad."*

BC: *"Where is your sister?"*

Fay: *"She is with my parents. They took her with them and left me with my nana. I haven't seen them since they left."*

BC: *"Can you recall the year or perhaps the country?"*

Fay: *"It's 1960 in England."*

Suddenly Fay got sad and I noticed that she was trying very hard not to cry.

BC: *"You seem sad. Why is that?"*

Fay: *"I am sad because I am not well. I have a cold... and something else. My feet are very heavy..."*

BC: *"Let's leave this scene as I want you to choose now what you want to recall."*

Fay: *"I am older now… maybe sixteen. I am in a school. I look very beautiful with my long hair. I wear it down. I don't like school, but I have to be there. My schoolmates are not very friendly. I know that they don't like me because I am different, but I don't know what is wrong with me."*

BC: *"Are your parents still away?"*

Fay: *"Yes. They never came back for me. I live with my grandmother."*

BC: *"Move again in time and experience another memory in the same lifetime."*

Fay: *"I am at home. I am seventeen now. My parents are back. My mother is very pretty."*

BC: *"Why did your parents come home?"*

Fay: *"Just to check up on me. They won't stay long. They will leave again. I am not sure where to. I have the feeling that they work in another country. It's not fair! And my legs are still so heavy!"*

I was sure by now that there was something wrong with Esme's legs and wondered if she was able to walk or if she actually had legs. I wanted to find out what was the cause of her *"heavy legs"*, so I instructed Fay to move to another moment in the same lifetime as Esme, hoping that things would come out.

Fay: *"I am eighteen now. I am in a dark room. I don't think that there is anybody around… but I am not sure about that. I may not be alone."*

BC: *"Do you know why you are there?"*

Fay: *"I was put there. Somebody put me there…"*

BC: *"Do you know who that may be?"*

Fay: *"Yes, my father locked me in there. I now see that I am not alone. My grandmother is with me. He locked us both in this room."*

BC: *"When you think about your father, would you be able to recognize him as somebody you know now?"*

Fay: *"Yes, he is familiar. He is somebody I met many years ago."*

BC: *"Do you know why you are locked in there?"*

Fay: *"My father doesn't want me around. My legs are very heavy... I am crawling."*

BC: *"Do you know why?"*

Tears started falling down her cheeks and Fay took a deep breath in before she answered.

Fay: *"I don't think that I have ever walked. I was injured when I was a baby. I never walked... I cannot walk."*

BC: *"Does your mother know that your father locked you in a room?"*

Fay: *"No... and she left. My father left too. I have to get out somehow."*

BC: *"Can your grandmother help?"*

Fay: *"No, she cannot."*

I suddenly started wondering whether her grandmother was alive or not. So I asked.

BC: *"Look at her please. Is she still alive?"*

Fay: *"I am not sure... maybe not."*

BC: *"Now focus on your father who locked you in that room and left. Is there something else he's done to you?"*

Fay: *"He hasn't hit me... just told me things. He said 'go away'. He doesn't want me because I cannot walk."*

BC: *"Do you remember your father's name?"*

Fay: *"Barry."*

BC: *"I want you now to recall the last minutes in this lifetime."*

Fay: *"I don't know where I am... maybe under the house. I was hiding there and couldn't get out. I was scared of something or somebody... maybe of my father. There is something right behind me. I feel cold. "*

BC: *"Do you know how old you are?"*

Fay: *"Eighteen... almost nineteen."*

BC: *"Do you know what happened?"*

Fay: *"I have broken bones... many broken bones... not enough air. I die there under the house."*

BC: *"Do you remember the lesson for that lifetime?"*

Fay: *"Yes. Hope. Hope is what keeps us alive."*

BC: *"Is there any energy you are carrying into the present, perhaps blocking your development?"*

Fay: *"Yes. Not being wanted. Not being loved. I am being told that. There are angels who show me a rainbow. Hope is precious, they say."*

I spent another good hour chatting with Fay after her regression. I remember that it was a beautiful summer afternoon and that she was my last client for the day. During the session, I heard rain drops on my window, but right after it, the rain stopped. I opened the window and noticed that the temperature had dropped a bit, which was quite nice.

I sat down and continue talking with Fay. I was curious about her thoughts with regards to what she just experienced. Fay seemed clearer... at least this was the first thing she said. She felt the pain of the little Esme not being able to walk and understood why she was different to any other children. She also sensed that her blockage in the present might have started in that past life as a little invalid girl.

I still keep in touch with Fay and see her from time to time and sometimes wonder if the fog over her life was lifted after the past life regression. What I know for sure is that the very delicate, soft and empathetic person she is changes her clients' lives. People like her are bright shining jewels.

We build our lives on expectations. We hope to succeed and we desire to be happy. We dream of positive outcomes every step of the way and, whilst that desire is still alive, it can heal the world.

You may have heard about the ancient Greek myth related to Pandora's box. The myth is based on the god Zeus, who created a box filled with evil spirits as revenge against Prometheus, who stole fire from him. When Pandora opened the box, anger, lust, revenge and greed were released to haunt humanity. Hope was the only spirit that stayed in the box. Pandora's box is just a myth, but I feel that behind it there is a seed of truth: hope can overcome every bad or unfortunate thing that affects us; it only needs to be released.

Hope is a main feature in many religions too. In Hinduism, for instance, hope is in charge of performing karmic rituals, whilst in Christianity it has the same value as faith and love, and refers to divine promises of afterlife for the chosen ones. However for Buddhism, hope is not essential and it is perceived in the same manner as desire is, just a less important phase in spiritual development.

I sometimes wonder if hope is an optimistic approach to reaching goals or a measure of naivety. It may be both at the end of the day, but what is essential is the level of endorphins that come with it, because hope, like the pleasure resulting from love, creates a state of excitement for what is to come. Therefore it focuses on the immediate and even far future while it also may create a positive vision of the present itself.

For the pessimistic, hope may be defined as seeing the future through rose tinted glasses. For the optimistic, it represents a certainty, influenced by them, others and - why not - the divine. Call me optimistic if you wish, but my hopes are connected to my goals and I will always be in a permanent hopeful state of mind to achieve them.

Karmic lesson 13

SACRIFICE

"We are all creatures of God"

I've never met a person like Trudy before. Her energy and joy-of-life are contagious. I first saw Trudy on a Monday evening and, right after she walked in the door, the room was filled with laughter and happiness. In her boho long white and pink dress, Trudy looked like a fairy. She wore her auburn hair down and the curls ran all over her face. She looked out of this world and I thought to myself that I wouldn't know what to pick first to cheer me up even more: her or a unicorn. She was positive, fun, full of life and a delight to have in my practice.

    She told me her whole life story in less than five minutes. Trudy was going through a divorce at the time, and the only one who was able to alleviate the stress caused by the separation was her boyfriend, a man she'd met just a few weeks ago. Then she talked about her teenage daughters, and every word she said was about the love she felt for them. I don't think she was capable of not liking somebody. Trudy was herself Love, all in capital letters.

    When I asked her why she felt that she needed a past life regression, Trudy started laughing and I found myself laughing with her. She was contagious indeed. Trudy believed that she required guidance regarding her future and her belief was that she could only find it in her past. I had to agree with her because I thought that this woman might know more than she let people see. Therefore I started inducing a hypnotic state and was prepared for whatever might come out.

Trudy: *"I am outdoors. There are big orange walls with some blue on them. I can see a little goat. I hear bells' sounds coming from far away."*

BC: *"Look at your feet and tell me if you see them."*

Trudy: *"I am a woman with smaller, delicate feet. They are darker."*

BC: *"Can you see what you are wearing?"*

Trudy: *"I am wearing a white muslin type dress. It is long and soft."*

BC: *"How old are you?"*

Trudy: *"I am in my twenties. My hair is dark, but I am not sure whether my eyes are brown or hazel. My skin is dark... golden dark."*

BC: *"Do you see any people around?"*

Trudy: *"I have the feeling that I am alone."*

BC: *"What is the year?"*

Trudy: *"It's 1694. I am in Morocco."*

BC: *"If there is nothing else that catches your attention, move to another scene that is significant for you."*

Trudy: *"I am in a breezy room. There is a baby boy with me... laughing. He may be nine months old. He's got green eyes. It feels like he is my daughter's baby."*

BC: *"How old are you now?"*

Trudy: *"I am sixty."*

BC: *"Do you recognize the daughter or her baby boy as being somebody you know in your present life?"*

Trudy: *"Yes, my daughter is one of my daughters now. I am not sure about the boy. He seems familiar, though..."*

BC: *"Is your daughter married?"*

Trudy: *"She is separated and I have to help her out with her son. I am on my own as well... because I don't think I can be loved... maybe I don't want to..."*

BC: *"That's fine. Is there anybody else you recognize in that life?"*

Trudy: *"Yes, there is that guy who keeps popping up. He has soft, dark facial hair and brown eyes. He is just a friend who helps us, but in a way he holds me back. He is my daughter's father in my life now."*

The sparkly Trudy became suddenly serious. I had the feeling that she was trying to work out how she felt.

BC: *"You seem sad. Why is that?"*

Trudy: *"I feel confusion... I don't know whether it is a sad life or I just make it sad."*

I noticed that Trudy couldn't recall more details about a life that she found rather sad. I felt overwhelmed seeing her crying, so I asked her to move to the very last few minutes in that lifetime. She started talking again, this time almost whispering.

Trudy: *"I am in a bed. I am ninety... I die of old age... There are lots of people there... but not quite there. I feel them but I am not able to see them. I am too old... but I see my grandson... not so little anymore. He is holding my hand. I am so proud of him. He has curly hair. Now that I look back, my life must have been more happy than sad."*

BC: *"That's good. What else do you see?"*

Trudy: *"I see myself leaving that body. I see angels. They tell me that it is OK to be here. They tell me that there was a contract with that man that kept me stuck for longer than needed. I don't know what they mean... but I understand what they want me to do. It's weird... I don't* know, but I do. Maybe he hurt me somehow... but it doesn't matter anymore."

BC: *"Do you remember your lesson in that lifetime?"*

Trudy: *"Yes. Give your time to others. Sacrifice your own time to help others... sacrifice."*

BC: *"Whenever you are ready, let your soul pick another body in another lifetime."*

Trudy: *"I am in a horse stable. I am a man now. I am in my thirties. I wear an apron."*

BC: *"What do you do in that stable?"*

Trudy. *"I think that I am doing horse shoes. It is very hot. There are scars on my arms."*

BC: *"Do you remember the country?"*

Trudy: *"England, but I don't remember the year."*

No matter how I formulated my questions, Trudy couldn't recall anything about the man she was in England, besides the horses and the heat in the stable. I knew that being stuck in a memory had happened to other clients before her. Some remembered more details later in the session; others refused to follow chronological order in a particular life they revisited. I sometimes believe that our subconscious may try to protect us from extremely dramatic memories. I thought that perhaps this was in Trudy's case too... but I was wrong. I was just preparing to guide her to another lifetime, when she suddenly started talking again.

Trudy: *"I am in an estate in America. I feel that I moved here... emigrated. There are a lot of black fences."*

BC: *"How old are you now?"*

Trudy: *"I am in my late thirties."*

BC: *"Do you have any family?"*

Trudy: *"I have a wife. She cooks well. She is lovely. We have two children, a seven year old boy and a five year old girl. They are both blonde. The girl's name is Louise. I don't remember the boy's name."*

BC: *"What else do you remember?"*

Trudy: *"I am well off, but it has been hard. I worked hard. I own a house with a garden and I see my property on the side of the garden. I do well."*

BC: *"What is your name?"*

Trudy: *"My name is Franz."*

BC: *"Do any of your wife or children's energies resemble somebody in the present?"*

Trudy: *"My wife is an old friend and my daughter is my daughter now."*

BC: *"Now find yourself older in that lifetime as I count from one to three... one... two... three..."*

Trudy: *"I am on a farm... my daughter's farm. She is in her mid twenties. She has a boyfriend. I don't like him."*

BC: *"Why is that?"*

Trudy: *"He wasn't very honest in the past. I recognize him. He is my boyfriend now. It's amazing how clearly I see that."*

BC: *"What about your son? How is he doing?"*

Trudy: *"He is traveling now... on a boat. He has a beautiful lady. Oh my goodness, I recognize her. She is a man I know now."*

BC: *"How is your wife doing?"*

Trudy: *"She is lovely. She loves gardening, cooks beautiful pies and cakes and looks very well after me."*

BC: *"Do you remember the year?"*

Trudy: *"1939."*

BC: *"Go now to the moment of your death and tell me what you see."*

Trudy: *"It seems to be quite brutal. It is dark. There are people around, but I don't know who they are. They want to hurt me. I have a sharp pain in my head. They probably hit me."*

BC: *"Do you know why?"*

Trudy: *"Because I was helping somebody. I was hiding someone... a man. That person is still alive. I saved him..."*

BC: *"Do you recognize any of the people who hurt you?"*

Trudy: *"Yes. One is my husband I am divorcing at the moment. I feel like I am leaving my body. I die on the ground. I see blood..."*

BC: *"That's fine. What do you see, hear or feel?"*

Trudy: *"I feel kind of angels around and a master angel... like a master over all angels... I hear a French horn."*

BC: *"Do you remember your lesson in that lifetime?*

Trudy: *"Sacrifice. Do what's right and save others. Don't hate people, love people, save people, and look after people... save people. We are all creatures of God."*

I was absolutely right about Trudy. No other client of mine summarized the whole Universe in just one sentence. *"We are all creatures of God"*. She said it as if it was not a big deal, but I knew that there was only one amazing Trudy and she, more than others, was able to understand the essence of all that we are. She was a fairy indeed.

I haven't seen Trudy since her past life regression, but I remember often her laughter and her joyful voice. I sometimes think about how fortunate the people in her life are, and, for an hour whilst the regression lasted, I was one of them.

Sacrifice has its etymology in the Latin word *"sacrificium"* which may have a religious meaning, because it refers to an act of animal sacrifice performed by priests as a religious ritual. You may have heard, or read about, animal sacrifice in ancient Greece, ancient Rome, Judaism and Hinduism. I've never encountered any reference to these rituals being part of Buddhism, perhaps because killing animals is contrary to their main principles.

In many ancient cultures worldwide though, human sacrifice was what apparently appealed to several gods people worshiped. I grew up reading appalling stories about the Aztec civilization and the importance of human sacrifice in their own belief system. I found them atrocious then and I am still disgusted now. However, for Christians thousands of years ago, animal sacrifice was a symbol of their hope regarding the afterlife. For them, the main human hecatomb, Jesus, was sacrificed to allow ultimate salvation and secure a place in the heavenly existence.

For me, sacrifice has a totally different meaning. Meeting people half way; compromising; 'giving in' when it is for the sake of others; acknowledging other people's feelings and acting upon them, are the ways I envision modern day sacrifice. In my opinion, giving up something for another person's happiness or even sometimes giving in, are easy sacrifices we can all make in the name of peace and harmony.

BRIGITTE CALLOWAY

Lesson 14

HARD WORK

"Don't overdo it"

Gloria attended many of the workshops I taught last year. Month by month, workshop by workshop, I used to see her face there. She even came for a group past life regression I held in one of the local halls. She never talked, she never asked questions and I put that down to her shyness. However, sometime last year, I approached her and our conversation bloomed. When the shyness disappeared, Gloria was smart and intelligent. She wasn't ordinary or less interested than others. She was delightful and a pleasure to be around.

In time, I started looking for her at each new workshop I taught; and she was always there. She was eager for knowledge and I thought to myself that her parents picked the right name for her because she was truly glorious.

Halfway through last year, Gloria and I started chatting on one of the social media channels and, as time passed, we became friends. Around the same time, she graduated from the graphic design course she had started a few years ago, whilst working full time. She told me that she wanted to open her own business, but at that moment in time she couldn't because, in order to pay her bills, she was forced to keep her job. I understood completely because I knew that Gloria was single after a long term relationship that had gone pear-shaped. Gloria had to work because there was nobody she could lean on.

I am always delighted when a friend asks for my services and, when Gloria wanted a past life regression, I booked her into the first available spot. She arrived for the appointment one Tuesday at lunchtime and I noticed that she was tired. She told me that she had recently been promoted to a management role and her responsibilities doubled overnight. She was calm and open to whatever the regression might have brought forward.

We chatted for a few minutes before she relaxed to the stage when she was able to start her journey in one of her past lives.

Gloria: *"It's dark, but I see purple-blue specks of color. I also see trees with big branches."*

BC: *"What trees do you see?"*

Gloria: *"Very tall trees with big branches. I feel that I am a child."*

BC: *"Can you see your feet?"*

Gloria: *"Yes. I am barefoot... the feet of a ten year old boy."*

BC: *"What can you remember about that child?"*

Gloria: *"I have blonde hair and blue eyes."*

BC: *"What are you doing where you are?"*

Gloria *"I am hunting."*

BC: *"What is your name?"*

Gloria: *"My name is George."*

BC: *"What are you wearing?"*

Gloria: *"I wear brown overalls... boy's overalls."*

BC: *"What can you remember about your parents?*

Gloria: *"I don't have parents. I don't know what happened to them. They are still around though. I know for sure that I am not an orphan. My auntie looks after me."*

BC: *"What is the year?"*

Gina: *"1820."*

BC: *"Do you remember where you are living?"*

Gloria: *"My home is in Prague."*

BC: *"Let's now move to another scene in the same lifetime as George and, when you are there, let me know."*

Gloria: *"I am nineteen now. I am outdoors somewhere."*

BC: *"Are you still living with your auntie?"*

Gloria: *"No. I am on my own. My auntie passed away. I am alone. I don't have a girlfriend either."*

BC: *"On your own at nineteen..."*

Gloria: *"Yes, I don't have anybody. I work as a bailer and I live in a kind of barn... very small barn. I am very poor."*

BC: *"That's fine. Do you have any friends?"*

Gloria: *"No friends... nobody."*

BC: *"If there is nothing else you can recall, move now to another scene in the same life as George."*

Gloria: *"I am on a boat... small boat. I am fishing. I am older now... I am twenty-nine."*

BC: *"Do you have a family of your own?"*

Gloria: *"Yes, I have a wife."*

BC: *"Can you recall her name?"*

Gloria: *"Her name is Rebecah."*

BC: *"Is she somebody you know in the present life?*

Gloria: *"Yes, she is very familiar. I know that she is somebody I've met. I really don't know who... Hmm... She is a colleague I work with now."*

BC: *"Do you have children?"*

Gloria: *"No, we don't have children."*

BC: *"Is it a happy life or a sad life?'*

Gloria: *"It's a sad life. It's too much work."*

BC: *"Is Rebecah sad too?"*

Gloria: *"Yes, she is.... She is very lonely. I work too much."*

BC: *"Are you still living in the same barn?"*

Gloria: *"No. We don't live in the barn anymore. We live in a hut."*

As she recalled her life in Prague, Gloria's face looked even more tired than she was when she arrived, and I felt truly sorry for her. I would have loved her to have remembered happier memories, but again, she was in charge with which lifetime she wanted to revisit.

BC: *"Move now another few years in time. Where are you now?"*

Gloria: *"I am on the streets... somewhere in Prague. I am fifty now."*

BC: *"What else do you remember?"*

Gloria: *"Rebecah is not alive anymore. She died of lung cancer. We haven't had children..."*

BC: *"Are you still working?"*

Gloria: *"No. I'm not. I couldn't work anymore. I am limping."*

BC: *"How did that happen?"*

Gloria: *"I was run over. I don't remember exactly how it happened."*

I noticed Gloria as she remembered her sad life as George. There was a level of calmness about her, she seemed at ease, and I knew that she accepted everything that came out in her regression. Then I looked out the window at the magnolia tree that was in bloom and I thought that peaceful moments like this are hard to forget.

BC: *"Go now to the last moments in that lifetime. How old are you now?"*

Gloria: *"Sixty-two... I am sitting somewhere. I am coughing blood."*

BC: *"So there is something wrong with your lungs."*

Gloria: *"Yes, I am sick. I see now white light. It looks like angels. I feel good. I am being told something, but don't hear clearly."*

BC: *"Do you remember the lesson for the life you just revisited?"*

Gloria: *"Work... You don't have to overwork. Don't overdo it. There are always opportunities."*

I felt sad as Gloria talked. The lifetime she remembered was not fun and I wondered what impact it might have had on her. Sometimes, when I listen to my clients' memories I am overwhelmed; other times their reminiscences bring tears to my eyes. It's no secret that some people have sad existences, whilst others seem truly blessed in every aspect of their lives. It is just the way it is!

Gloria seemed at peace with what she recalled though, perhaps because she was now able to draw a line between the effects of what hard work would have had on George in comparison to her present life. Gloria loved being active and, as tired as she may have been, she never complained. As I talked with her, I understood how stubborn she was in making sure she did a good job. She was meticulous and nothing could stop her when it came to her work. I knew that opening her own business might have been an unaccomplished dream, but looking deep into her eyes, I understood that the first step in reaching it started in the moment she remembered her life as George.

The effort we put into our jobs is different for each person. For some, work comes naturally whilst others struggle to deliver results in their everyday career. I don't know what work is for you, but for me it is excitement and a way of keeping myself active. It may be because I do what I love for a living or perhaps because I have a productive nature. However, there should be a balance between earning a living and 'doing' a living. It may be easier said than done for those who need two - or even three - jobs to sustain themselves and provide for their families, but even they should find equilibrium. Life can be taught to some, I agree, but in most cases it is as we do it.

People work for a living now, and they worked in the ancient past, when bartering was the only system of exchanging products. It may have been easier then, you may think, but the truth is that people still needed to put time and effort into what they had to do for a living. I always wondered if introducing money into trading products changed everything in human lives, but a form of paying for the essentials has been around forever. No one knows for sure who invented money, but history proves that clay tokens, an equivalent of monetary redeemable proofs, was present in ancient Egypt, whilst Romans used bronze coins.

I was taught in school that Phoenicians were involved in the first modern monetary system, but, to be perfectly honest, I haven't found any evidence that the copper coins used then might have been the very first ones. What is, however, a certainty is the fact that the famous disciple of Socrates, Plato, believed that coins used in exchange for products should not have been made out of precious metals such as gold or silver. Plato believed that these metals already had a value of their own, independent from the coins' value itself. The ancient Greek philosopher Aristotle opposed Plato's *"carthalist theory"*, apparently with more success because precious and semiprecious coins were used in trading for centuries.

We work for the benefits earned money can give us. Some need more money; others need less. Some work to survive; others for pleasure. I am not sure what your situation is, but in my case work and pleasure are in symbiosis; I enjoy my work and the effects it has on other people - and me. I may be one of the lucky ones or I may just target the fortune and fate myself.

Karmic lesson 15
CHANGE

"Ups and downs"

Marie is a statuesque woman; one of those gorgeous people you usually only see on the television. When she arrived one early evening in November wearing a striped dress, my first thought was that one had to have a body like hers to be able to get away with horizontal stripes. With pale skin and very long blonde hair, curled at the ends, Marie was a beautiful woman indeed. She looked even more astonishing when she started speaking. Her gentleness and softness suddenly came out with each word she said.

Usually my clients find me through word-of-mouth. Not Marie though. She felt that a past life regression was needed at that stage in her life, so she researched on the Internet with the aim of locating a practitioner. When a client finds me through my website, I know that the desire to be regressed is even deeper than for one who hears about me in their social circle and, out of curiosity, decides to go through hypnosis. Marie knew what she wanted and looked for the person who could deliver.

What usually interests me is the reason why a client decides to be regressed. For Marie it was an inexplicable fear of something happening to her children. She was protective and there was nothing wrong with that, but, in her case, her accentuated fear created an anxiety that rose up anytime one of her children was out of her sight.

While I started relaxing her by talking about beautiful secluded beaches, I heard my husband in the garden talking to our neighbor. I couldn't discern any words, but I recognized their voices.

Marie: *"It's quiet. I see the sunset."*

BC: *"I want you now to look down at your feet."*

Marie: *"They are whiter. I am wearing sandals."*

BC: *"What color are your sandals?"*

Marie: *"Brown with buckles on the sides."*

BC: *"Are you a woman or a man?"*

Marie: *"I am a woman. I wear a whitish colored dress... no pattern on it... harsh fabric... just passed my knees."*

BC: *"How old do you feel you are?"*

Marie: *"I feel like a young woman. I think that I am eighteen."*

BC: *"Do you feel happy or sad?"*

Marie: *"Very sad. I am walking on a dusty road. I don't feel comfortable. I don't see people around, but I know that they are hiding somewhere behind the road. They are not friendly. They are dangerous..."*

BC: *"What else do you remember about yourself?"*

Marie: *"I am ugly. Everything about me is ugly... nothing beautiful. I am alone. I don't have any family."*

BC: *"Ugly?"*

Marie: *"Yes. There is something that is not right. I am not a pretty girl."*

That came as a surprise actually because I couldn't imagine this stunning woman being ugly... not even in a past life!

BC: *"Tell me what happens."*

Marie: *"This road is dangerous and I feel scared. It's dusty. I feel that I won't make it if I keep walking, but I have to go home and this is the only way. I almost see my house. There is a light in the window. I know how my house looks inside. There is an old chair I love... like a recliner type. I remember the chair very well. And there are three brown cushions I remember."*

Marie started shaking on my recliner and I knew that what she was remembering was related to a traumatic experience. I waited a while before she talked again, but instead of sharing her memories about the girl on a dusty road, she jumped to another life; so I understood that her life might have ended on that dusty road.

Marie: *"I can see that I wear brown shoes and long black trousers."*

BC: *"Are you a woman or a man?"*

Marie: *"I am a man... a forty year old man. I am a blacksmith."*

BC: *"Do you know where you live?"*

Marie: *"I am a Jewish man, living in Poland, in 1739."*

BC: *"What is your name?"*

Marie: *"It sounds like Aaron... hmm... I am pretty sure that Aaron is my name."*

BC: *"Do you remember your family?"*

Marie: *"Yes. I have a wife. Her name is Rachel."*

BC: *"Do you remember her being somebody you know in the present life?"*

Marie: *"Yes, she is my daughter now."*

BC: *"Do you have any children?"*

Marie: *"Yes, a girl and a boy. The girl is six and the boy is eight years old. I don't remember my daughter's name... maybe Ruth. My son is Abraham."*

BC: *"Are any of them somebody in your present life?"*

Marie: *"My daughter is my son now."*

BC: *"Tell me what else you can recall."*

Marie: *"We are poor, but we have a roof over our heads. We are at peace with our lives and happy that we found a way of surviving. We have faith. I work hard to put food on the table. My family is happy."*

BC: *"Tell me about your home."*

Marie: *"It's not a big house. Everything looks brown. I hear my son Abraham talking. He is at the table. My wife is cooking in the kitchen."*

BC: *"What else happens?"*

Suddenly, Marie panicked as she remembered something that made her uncomfortable. A few minutes later, she started crying silently.

Marie: *"Something bad happens. My daughter is missing. Something happened... something... maybe a fire. I think she is gone. My wife is concerned. I hear a big noise... fire. It's like we are all gone."*

BC: *"Just float above the scene if you feel anxious and tell me if there is something else you see."*

Marie: *"Peaceful... I am loved."*

I knew that her soul left the body of the Jewish man she was.

BC: *"Can you remember what was the lesson for the life you recalled?"*

Marie: *"Change! From good to bad there is only a second... ups and downs... change!"*

BC: *"Is there any dishonored promise or contract you may carry in the current life?"*

Marie *"I promised to take care of my children. I couldn't save them... it breaks my heart."*

Marie opened her eyes but took her time to speak again. The regression was nothing like she expected it to be, she said with a soft velvety voice. She told me that on the way to my practice she anticipated that she wouldn't remember anything, but the dramatic memories she recalled made her think about what else was possible. She booked a second appointment just before she left. Once I closed the door behind her, I watched her walking towards her car. In front of my eyes, everything was alluring: purple-blue hydrangeas, ivory roses, tall ferns and this beautiful woman who fitted perfectly into nature's glory.

We alter every day according to the situations life throws at us. Life is a process of natural selection, in which we have to adapt and transform. We change ourselves, move homes, get over passions and we try to modify people, ignoring that 'each is to their own'. Sometimes the process of changing is soft and gentle; other times traumatic adjustments are required. At the end of the day it is about how we adapt to the whole process of changing rather than why we aim to modify our lives.

You may have heard about transformational changes, mostly used in business organizational processes; or even transitional changes, in the same environment. People change very similarly to the alterations made during these. Some change for the better; others for worse, depending on the initial intent and the strategies used.

Each modification brings new alternatives and a brand new perspective on life. We can control our own transformation, but cannot govern the world changing around us. Sometimes we make rigid changes to our circumstances, appearance and behavior; other times we are more flexible in our approach.

If we focus on personal transformation, the effect is ultimately metamorphosis of who, where and what we are. Everything should therefore relate to what the famous Indian activist Mahatma Gandhi once said: *"Be the change you want to see in the world"*.

BRIGITTE CALLOWAY

Karmic lesson 16
INDEPENDENCE

"Know how to survive"

Jimmy rang me right after he read my book *"You have lived many times"*, lent to him by one of his mates. It was very late one Saturday evening and I negotiated with myself whether or not to take the call. I did, and he started talking about my book and how reading it had given him the urge to go through a regression himself. A week later, Jimmy was in my practice, ready to remember his past.

Jimmy is a tall 'man's man' in his late fifties. Right after meeting him, I noticed that there was a kind of roughness about him. His answers to my initial questions were statements about himself, the world and the whole Universe and he seemed to be strongly opinionated about everything he knew, or thought he knew. However, once I started figuring him out more clearly, I realized that he was a gentle man with a vast life experience and that he actually knew what he was talking about.

When he felt comfortable with sharing even more about his life, Jimmy talked about his farm, his wife - who he definitely adored - and his grown up children, now living overseas; about his university studies in a subject that had nothing to do with farming and his dream of traveling the world. He told me with a sense of embarrassment that he has never been on a plane and always wondered how that might feel. Instead of travelling, he'd worked hard his whole life and built an enviable fortune, and lately he'd thought of selling the business and packing up for a few years' world trip.

While inducing trance, I had no clue what answers Jimmy wanted to get from revisiting past lives. I however understood for sure that this guy would enjoy the world, once he started discovering it.

Jimmy: *"I feel that I am a young girl, wearing a long rough dress with a warm wool sweater on top. I feel the texture of the dress rubbing against my legs."*

BC: *"Do you know how old you may be?"*

Jimmy: *"Nineteen... almost twenty."*

BC: *"What else do you remember about yourself?"*

Jimmy: *"My name is Ana. I have long hair, plaited just behind my ears. My hair is soft."*

BC: *"What color is your hair?"*

Jimmy: *"I wouldn't know that because I cannot see. I am blind. I feel that I could see a little bit when I was a young girl, but cannot remember how much I was able to."*

Listening to Jimmy, I realized that I would have to carefully pick my questions because he remembered a life in which he suffered a visual impairment, so I decided to refer to his feelings instead, with regards to what he could recall.

BC: *"Where do you feel you may be at the moment?"*

Jimmy: *"I am in my own home. I know every corner of my house. I use a wooden stick when I walk. I feel that my father made it for me."*

BC: *"Is your father with you now?"*

Jimmy: *"No. Both my parents died last year and I am on my own. I have a brother who helps me sometimes, but he lives in another village... Hmm... We live in Russia. He is married and has a baby boy... He wanted me to move in with him, but I like it in my old parents' house."*

BC: *"Do you recognize your brother's energy?"*

Jimmy: *"He is my wife now."*

BC: *"So tell me how you manage to live on your own if you are blind."*

Jimmy: *"There is a neighbor, a kind woman who brings me food, but I am able to cook simple things too. I wash my clothes by hand and know how to hang out my washing. There is a friend who spends a few hours a day helping me out with domestic chores... he is a friend of mine."*

BC: *"Do you remember his name?"*

Jimmy: *"Ruben. He lives in the same village... very good friend."*

BC: *"Do you recognize him?"*

Jimmy: *"He is my uncle now."*

BC: *"Do you remember the year?"*

Jimmy: *"1721."*

BC: *"I want you now to remember memories from the same life, perhaps when Ana was a few years older."*

Jimmy: *"I am thirty-nine now. Ruben died and I am alone again."*

BC: *"What happened?"*

Jimmy: *"Ruben and I got married and he was a good man to me. There was no wedding... just between us... He was a builder and made many of the houses in the village. He put aside money for us. He was a good man... Then he died in a fire. He tried to save somebody's child when the house caught on fire... and he didn't make it out."*

BC: *"So how are you managing?"*

Jimmy: *"I don't have any problems. I know how to survive and Ruben left me with money. I buy products from my neighbors and can cook my meals. I can wash my clothes... There is a young girl who helps with cleaning...*

but the rest is fine. I feel lonely without my husband, but this is life! I go to church every Sunday... it's not far, just a few minutes away. I believe in God and God takes good care of me."

BC: "If there is nothing else you remember, go to the moment of your death and tell me what happens."

Jimmy: "I am a few years older... fifty-two maybe. I fell and broke a leg. The pain is horrible. The doctor said that it is infected. I die of that. My brother is here with me."

BC: "Anything else?"

Jimmy: "I feel very light and I can see now. I hear voices and there are colors... I think that there are colors. I blink because they hurt my eyes."

BC: "Do you remember the lesson you learnt as blind Ana?"

Jimmy: "Freedom... independence. Be prepared to break free. Know how to survive."

We didn't speak a lot after the regression. Maybe just a few words... I assumed that Jimmy might have felt speechless actually seeing himself in a woman's body. In most cases, clients expect to revisit a life of big fortune, wealth and perfect health. The strong Jimmy however remembered being a blind woman, who lost her husband early in life and lived in solitude. So when Jimmy left my practice, I wondered what the past life he revisited might have taught him.

Since then, I've received a couple of emails from him, mostly keeping me updated with his progress. Jimmy seemed happy managing his farm and enjoying time with his wife. Recently though I heard from a friend who knows him, that his farm was just about to be listed on the market this summer. My buddy also said that one of Jimmy's employees might buy it. I smiled when I heard the news and my friend asked me what was so funny. I kept smiling, but didn't answer him... I couldn't share how happy I was envisioning Jimmy on a plane traveling from place to place. It was between Jimmy and me!

History proves that countries went through wars in the desire for independence, and rivers of blood were required in the process of gaining it. Similarly, we humans want to break free from bad habits, dominating relationships or even old lives and sometimes sacrifices have to be made. We want to be in charge of our own destiny and aim to stand up tall and make our statements loud and clear in our own way. That doesn't mean for a second that we would want to become an enclave ruling an isolated non-social existence.

Fear and independence don't make a good couple. Through association, I remember one of my dear friends who was in an abusive relationship a few years ago, and confided in us girls that her only desire was to leave the man and start a new life. *"I want to break free"*, she used to tell us anytime we got together. Then she shared her fears with regards to how she would be able to maintain her existence without him and provide for herself. She had no children, so there was no extra mouth to feed, and no cat or dog she was responsible for. We, her friends, heard the same old story all over again for years. She is still in the same dominating relationship because of her fear of self-governing her life. Like her, many others might want to make changes to their lives, but the panic of having to actually think for themselves stops the process before it's even started.

There is nothing more beautiful than courageous, independent people, in charge of their own lives. One can choose to be that or one can live the way they always have, repeating the same mistakes and giving up their power. It is just a matter of choice!

Karmic lesson 17

COURAGE

"You can save lives"

Paul came in for his appointment straight from work, wearing denim shorts, a blue stained T-Shirt with a small logo on the chest and builder's brown boots. He left the boots in front of my door and shook my hand firmly. Paul sat down on the recliner whilst looking straight into my eyes. Then he waited for me to speak first.

I explained about the whole process and gave him the forms to fill in. When I asked for more details about him, he said that he was a self-employed builder with loads of contracts in the area. I already guessed that he worked outdoors because he was very tanned, but let him talk further. Then he spoke about his guitar and his passion for music. Paul was a guitar player and everyday after work he rehearsed in his garage with some friends. They formed a band and had occasional gigs in the city.

Then Paul began explaining how awful it would be not being able to work and play his guitar and, to be perfectly honest, I found that quite odd. He seemed in good shape and couldn't understand what he was afraid of. So I asked. Paul kept silent for a few minutes and then he told me about the nightmares he'd had lately about losing his arms. Now that I knew the reason that brought him in, I was ready to start the session by guiding him to the enigmatic world of hypnosis.

Suddenly, I realized I had no clue how old he was, so I looked at the forms he completed and left on my desk. Thirty-six years old, I read whilst clearing my voice. He looked younger than that, I thought to myself. In the meantime Paul was so relaxed and ready to discover his soul's journey in past lives.

Paul: *"I am a young black boy. I don't look older that six. I live in a weird clay building. It looks like an igloo, but it is made of mud and straw. It is crowded in my little home because I have a brother and my grandfather living with us."*

BC: *"What about your parents?"*

Paul: *"I am not sure. I was never told. All I know is what my grandfather said about that."*

BC: *"What did he say?"*

Paul: *"All sorts of stories, mostly that they died in a sort of epidemic."*

BC: *"Tell me more about you."*

Paul: *"I am somewhere in South America. I know the country, but don't really remember its name."*

BC: *"No worries. Do you know the year?"*

Paul: *"Very, very long time ago... six hundred or seven hundred years ago maybe..."*

BC: *"So what do you do?"*

Paul: *"I help my grandfather. He is the shaman of the village. He mixes all sorts of leaves and makes medicines. He can treat everything. The gods tell him how to do it."*

BC: *"How do you help him?"*

Paul: *"I know every ingredient and I know how to mix them. I need to be careful when I pick grasses and leaves... some are poisonous."*

BC: *"Is your grandfather somebody you know in the present?"*

Paul: *"My girlfriend."*

Remembering his girlfriend, Paul smiled gently and my first thought was that she must be very special.

BC: *"Do you know your name?"*

Paul: *"It sounds like Arao."*

I instructed Paul to move a few years later and was curious to hear more about the young South-American grandson of a shaman.

Paul: *"I am twelve now. My grandfather is very sick and I am the one to be in charge... not as a shaman... just giving people the potions he prepared. I need to do something... otherwise my grandfather will die."*

BC: *"What can you do?"*

Paul: *"There is a berry... or something like a berry... that can heal everything. I may have to go and get it... but it is very far away and I don't know the way. My grandfather said that it is three days walk away. He doesn't let me go... I am far too young for a trip like that."*

BC: *"Move now to another moment in the same lifetime as Arao."*

Paul: *"Many people are sick in the village. They all have what my grandfather has. Their bodies are swollen and have boils on their skins. Something has to be done. My grandfather is worse now."*

BC: *"Are you sick too?"*

Paul: *"No. I am well, but people are dying... babies and young children."*

BC: *"Don't stop. Tell me more."*

Paul: *"I take some water and start walking. I have to find the berry my grandfather told me about. He doesn't know the way there... he just knows about it. His grandfather told him stories about the place that berry bush grows."*

BC: *"Does he know you are going?"*

Paul: *"He wouldn't let me go."*

BC: *"Tell me about your trip."*

Paul: *"I walk and walk... The sun goes down... I stop to sleep on the grass... then I walk again.... There are rocks I have to climb. My feet are bleeding and I have blisters on my palms. It is very hot and I don't have any water left."*

BC: *"Are you still walking?"*

Paul: *"Yes... for days. I am up somewhere on a green platform. I remember what my grandfather said about the place. I think that I may be close to it. The sun is burning..."*

BC: *"Do you find the berry?"*

Paul: *"Yes... it's like a bush with very sharp pins. The berries are a purple color. I picked them all! I have to find some water... I am thirsty and my lips are bleeding."*

BC: *"Do you get back to the village in time?"*

Paul: *"Yes, only just. I am very tired and run down. Many people have died since I left and the village smells of death... I mix the berries with some special leaves... then add water... hmm... yes, water."*

BC: *"Is your grandfather still alive?"*

Paul: *"Yes, but he is very ill. I don't know if he's going to make it."*

BC: *"Tell me what happens."*

Paul: *"I go to every home and take them potions to drink and rub on their bodies. Some people get better... others still die. I have the feeling that the epidemic stopped spreading but only strong bodies would make it. My grandfather gets better, but he is weak. He is the oldest one to survive."*

BC: *"Go now to a memory you can recall from a few days later and tell me what you see."*

Paul: *"It's morning. The village is waking up. People are healed... We have to get rid of the dead bodies. People celebrate... They call my name... they are grateful. My grandfather is there... still weak, but so much better."*

BC: *"Leave this memory behind and move to another one that is significant for that lifetime."*

Paul: *"I am twenty now... attending a ceremony. It's beautiful! People are happy... I am happy. I am their new leader now... I didn't expect that... but they trust me. I saved the village and they believe that I was compassionate and... willing to help. I am fair and fearless... I am a kind of chief of the village. My grandfather is so proud. He is still the shaman and I still help him."*

BC: *"Is there any young woman in your life?"*

Paul: *"There is a girl I will marry today in the same ceremony. I don't remember her name, but I know that it sounds pretty similar to mine... maybe starting with 'A'"*

BC: *"Is she somebody you recognize?"*

Paul: *"She is my brother now."*

Paul smiled, and then started speaking again. I realized that he jumped in time to another happy moment.

Paul: *"I am old, surrounded by children and grandchildren. We sit on the ground and eat our food. I am still the chief and the village is happy... no illness, no worries... I wish my grandfather could see how proud I am. He died a long time ago. He was old. We have a new shaman. It is one of my sons."*

BC: *"Is he somebody in your present life?"*

Paul: *"Oh yes. He is my mother."*

Paul then shared with me memories about his death in the lifetime as Arao, a South American courageous chief.

Paul: *"I am very old... ready to go. I don't see very well and I barely can move. I had a good life, but the time has come for me to go to our gods. I hear people singing outside... my people celebrating my life... I am going to heaven."*

BC: *"Do you remember what your lesson was to learn in the lifetime you remembered?"*

Paul: *"Yes. Courage was my lesson. Don't be afraid! You can save lives. I fulfilled my mission. I saved a village. What an awesome life!"*

Paul opened his eyes and smiled. He was as calm as when he first came in. I let him talk for a few minutes and then asked if the regression helped diminish the fear he had. This was the moment when he became excited. He said that he found himself so connected to his soul's incarnation as a South American fearless boy who became the chief of his tribe. As I looked at him, I understood that deep down he was a courageous man who had lost hope for a while.

I keep in touch with Paul sporadically. To be perfectly honest, it is he who texts from time to time sending me short videos from his gigs. He knows I love music too. His first text came a week after the regression. It was short: *"I trusted you because you play drums".* I started laughing as I remembered that on the long corridor, on his way to my practice room, Paul would have seen my drum kit. Sometimes the rapport I build with my clients has nothing to do with what I was taught. No hypnotherapy manual states that a musical instrument may be the best way to connect with a client.

Fearlessness is a quality not many people possess because of the many fears and phobias we accumulate during our lives. Courage incorporates a level of bravery that, if it's not taken to the extreme, can successfully help us overcome any obstacles.

More than ten years ago, there was a dangerous game of so-called *"courage"*, very popular in the youngsters' groups here in New Zealand. I am not sure whether it was something branded here or if these kids borrowed it from similar groups overseas. The game was called *"playing chicken"* and involved actually risking their lives by standing still on a high speed segment of a street, waiting for cars to get closer. They then had to jump out of the way when a car got just a couple of meters away from them. To be honest, it was the most stupid game I have ever heard of, equally idiotic as Russian roulette. Anyway, after a few fatal accidents, the game faded away. These kids thought that nothing could scare them, but, to be perfectly honest, this has nothing whatsoever to do with courage. This was just a useless form of bravery that didn't help anybody.

Courage is a calculated risk that involves determination and even endurance. Courage has an effect that in most cases is positive. Just remember the heroes whose names stayed alive over centuries. Their courage saved lives and encouraged others to pass through hard times. This is the type of bravery we are in need of. These are the people who can change and rule the world.

Karmic lesson 18
LOYALTY

"If you are loyal to people, they are loyal to you"

Of all my clients, I remember Shirley the most because I assessed her on my birthday. I usually take my birthdays off, but last year I booked an assessment by mistake and, when I realized my error, it was too late to cancel.

Shirley arrived right on time and while talking with her, all I could think of was the lunch I planned to have in my favorite cafe, at one of the garden centers in the city. The conversation was truly pleasant and I had a feeling that Shirley would become more than a client in the future. For the time being however, I went through the procedures required to build rapport and know more about my client.

Shirley and I are very similar, both around the same age, both in our second marriages... both blondes. From the moment she walked in, I liked her instantly; friendship at first sight perhaps... I liked the fact that she was a career woman and a very dedicated mother. On the other hand, she looked awesome in her white trousers and very sophisticated baby-blue silk top when I first met her.

Shirley had charisma and the determination of a lioness. As I have said, she is awesome!

Shirley approached me for classical hypnotherapy and booked three sessions on the spot, and six weeks later, after the treatment ended, she rang and booked another three sessions for a totally different problem she wanted sorted. She did, however, request that the last session would be a past life regression, sometime in November. I am still not sure whether she booked a regression based on curiosity or a feeling that she really needed it, but I knew that this whole new experience would have helped her understand more about herself.

It was a sunny day when Shirley came in for her regression wearing a beautiful summery turquoise dress. The color worked perfectly with her olive complexion. By then, I knew Shirley very well and she was comfortable with me too. Without any introduction, I started inducing hypnosis and Shirley went under fast.

BC: *"What do you see, hear or feel?"*

Shirley: *"I am a girl. I am barefoot and wear ankle length pants... grey pants."*

BC: *"What else do you know about yourself?"*

Shirley: *"I have blonde hair and my skin is fair."*

BC: *"How old are you?"*

Shirley: *"Mid teens... seventeen?"*

I smiled noticing that she actually asked approval for the age she remembered she was.

BC: *"Do you know where you are?"*

Shirley: *"I am in a castle in England... a very big castle with many rooms. The walls are made of rocks. It's stunning."*

BC: *"Can you recall the year?"*

Shirley: *"Yes. 1300."*

BC: *"So what are you doing in that big castle in the 1300s in England?"*

Shirley: *"I am hiding. I am supposed to be working. I believe that I work as a servant for the lady of the castle. I escaped."*

BC: *"Why is that?"*

Shirley: *"She is very good to me. She is just a young lady, married to a very harsh man. I think that I am hiding from her husband's people."*

BC: *"Do you recognize her energy?"*

Shirley: *"She is my cousin now."*

BC: *"Do you have any family?"*

Shirley: *"I have parents. I don't have a good feeling about them. They work for the castle's owners too, but they are hungry and sick. I don't think that they will live for much longer."*

BC: *"Do you remember your name?"*

Shirley: *"Yes. My name is Elisha."*

BC: *"Tell me about your chores in the castle."*

Shirley: *"I help the lady dress and I am her confidant. Her husband is mean and suspects that she is cheating on him."*

BC: *"Is she?"*

Shirley: *"No, she is not, but she plans to run away. I help her... She is a foreigner, born in Scotland. She speaks funny."*

BC: *"How do you help her?"*

Shirley: *"I talk with people she trusts. She will run away in a few days. I will go with her. We then will go back to her parents' castle."*

BC: *"Can you recall her name?"*

Shirley: *"Magdalene."*

BC: *"Move to another scene in the same life as Elisha. Let me know when you are there."*

Shirley: *"I am sitting at the table. There are many people around me. I am still in the castle. I feel that I eat dinner with the masters. My lady is next to me... we don't speak a lot."*

BC: *"Do you feel happy or sad?"*

Shirley: *"I am happy when I am around people. My lady loves me and I am privileged."*

BC: *"Do you recognize anybody?"*

Shirley: *"Some of the people there are friends now... hmm... the master is my ex husband."*

BC: *"What happens next?"*

Shirley: *"Nothing much. We eat. The master is drunk... other people are drunk too. They laugh and speak loudly. My lady and I just look at each other. We will leave very soon... I will have such a good life in Scotland..."*

BC: *"I want you now to remember the memory of you escaping the castle if that happened."*

Shirley blushed suddenly and started being restless like the escape was happening in this very moment.

Shirley: *"We ride horses... I don't see their colors because it is very dark. We have to meet some people who will help us further."*

BC: *"Do they?"*

Shirley: *"Yes. We travel further. It's so cold and dark... I feel that it's raining."*

BC: *"Do you arrive safely?"*

Shirley: *"Yes, we do. Life is good now. I am so loved and I am more of a friend than a servant... they gave me a nice room."*

BC: *"Move now to the last minutes in that lifetime and tell me what happens."*

Shirley: *"I am falling from a cliff."*

BC: *"How did you get there?"*

Shirley: *"I am not sure, but I remember wandering around."*

BC: *"Do you think that you have been pushed?"*

Shirley: *"No. It was an accident."*

BC: *"How old are you now?"*

Shirley: *"Not quite twenty yet."*

BC: *"Are there people around you?"*

Shirley: *"Yes, my friend, and some of her guests. They witness everything. There is nothing they can do."*

BC: *"Was there any contract or promise you made in that lifetime that you may have carried into the present?"*

Shirley: *"I promised Magdalene to always be with her. She has to manage on her own now..."*

BC: *"Was it a happy or a sad life?"*

Shirley: *"It started off sad, but then it was great. I was a servant and lived like a lady. I had a great life! It was short though... shame!"*

BC: *"Do you remember the lesson Elisha had to learn?"*

Shirley: *"I had to learn about loyalty... saving a life by being faithful. If you are loyal to people, they are loyal to you... maybe."*

The lessons my clients remember learning in past lives fascinate me. To be perfectly honest, the whole process of recalling experiences from other existences is mesmerizing as well as the memories themselves. In Shirley's case, loyalty is one of the values that seem more and more lost nowadays, when most relationships are not necessarily based on fidelity. Perhaps being disloyal or unfaithful is just a trend, or maybe some values have faded or even disappeared over time. Shirley however brought back, for me at least, the beauty of loyalty.

I keep in touch with Shirley and there is a sort of friendship that blossomed once my services for her finished. We don't find it necessary to see each other often, and we couldn't anyway because of our busy lifestyles. We are however what I would call each other's biggest fans. She recommended me to many of her friends and I had a wave of people coming from her immediate circle. That makes me think that I might have done something right. I, on the other hand, watch and applaud her accomplishments and mostly her more recent desire to travel. I put that down to her regression and I sometimes think that recalling a life when she died young, may have opened Shirley's eyes with regards to how fragile life is. Whatever it was, Shirley's photos from overseas are proof that she is happy and ultimately this is the only thing that matters.

When we refer to loyalty, the first thought that comes to mind may be related to relationships, mostly romantic ones. Perhaps fidelity and allegiance could have an emotional belonging. Loyalty has many facets though. There is a faith and devotion to a certain belief, in most cases a religious one; there is patriotism and then there is adherence with regards to a group. However, we mostly use loyalty when and how it serves us and blame our infidelity on circumstances and sometimes on other people. We have blind faith in our sport teams, but we break in a blink of an eye commitments and vows in relationships. We change our object of devotion based on what makes us happy in the moment. We tend to forget what we promised or we get bored of the commitments we made. In the name of happiness, we protect and we hurt people!

Most of us forget however that we have to be loyal to ourselves before we can be to others. Practicing trust in ourselves first helps us to develop the same behaviors with others. Being true to ourselves starts with knowing every aspect of our own behavior. There is no need to worship ourselves and there is no narcissism in discovering every detail of who we are.

Probably the best example with regards to loyalty is related to our pets. For them, there is a level of sacrifice, based on recognizing us as companions, providers and masters. Their devotion has no limits. I don't think that I have encountered the same behavior in humans as I have in pets. I remember a few years ago, when I broke my ankle and then, after surgery, I had to stay in bed for a few weeks. That was the time when I felt that my beloved dog Hendrix went through the same pain. He stood down at my feet for days, which was quite unusual for an energetic furry friend like him, and when I hopped around the house using my crutches to prevent my injured leg touching the ground, he followed me around with a kind of worry on his brave face. There was such a difference between his behavior and the conduct of most people I knew. If we could only learn from our pets what love and loyalty means!

Karmic lesson 19

DECISIVENESS

"Decide on the spot"

My county is famous in New Zealand for prosperous farms, so if you ever visit here, all you would see in between two towns or villages are beautiful cattle. Anyone who has a farm here in Taranaki, could secure a good retirement if they put in the effort and dedicate long hours to maintain and grow their business. I've had many farming clients in the past and enjoyed working with them. They were all decent, honest, hard working people. I wasn't surprised therefore when Peter asked for an appointment.

Peter is a farmer himself. In his late thirties, he is a tall, handsome guy, who feels in his element when he is outdoors. I have to admit that, based on his look, I expected him to have a strong voice; but he didn't. Peter was gentle and the tone of his voice was pure velvet. The conversation we had was out of the ordinary because Peter had a literate, intellectual way of expressing himself. Very well read, a university graduate, he was a delight to chat to.

As he talked about his life, I thought to myself that the gods were very generous with this guy. He was handsome, smart and very pleasant. He had a perfectly groomed ebony beard, very short dark hair and dark eyes. Despite his great personality and very appealing presence, Peter was single and there was no queue of potential partners at this front door. He however wanted a family and put his bachelor status down to a lack of time. Oh well, as I have said, farmers do indeed have a shortage of time off.

When I started instigating hypnosis, I thought that this session would be like every other I had conducted in the past. I was wrong though.

Peter: *"I am in the middle of the ocean... in the water."*

BC: *"How far away from the land?"*

Peter: *"Very far away... no way I can get back there."*

BC: *"What are you wearing?"*

Peter: *"A dress... hmm... but I don't think that I am a woman though."*

BC: *"How did you end up in the water?"*

Peter: *"I am not sure. I was on the boat. I haven't jumped."*

BC: *"Were you pushed?"*

Peter: *"Maybe..."*

BC: *"Do you see the boat?"*

Peter: *"No. It's gone... gone."*

BC: *"Is there anybody around you?"*

Peter: *"No. I am alone."*

Instantly Peter started looking around. His head moved from one side to the other like he was searching for somebody or something, while still keeping his eyes closed. At some stage he stopped and my first thought was that there might have been something that caught his attention. His whole body began suddenly shaking and I realized that he had seen something that scared him terribly. He made a weird noise and I understood that his life in that past existence finished. He may have been attacked or just sank. He kept silent for another few moments before he talked again.

Peter: *"I am a man of forty years old."*
BC: *"Where do you think you are?"*
Peter: *"Somewhere outdoors. It looks like a big piece of land... a farm."*
BC: *"Do you know where this farm may be?"*
Peter: *"It's in England."*
BC: *"Do you remember the year?*
Peter: *"Yes. It's 1782."*
BC: *"Does this farm belong to you?"*
Peter: *"No. It is in the family. It belongs to my family... not my immediate family though... not my parent's farm."*
BC: *"Do you remember your parents?"*
Peter: *"Very well."*
BC: *"Do they feel like being somebody you know in the present?"*
Peter: *"They are my parents now."*
BC: *"Do you have siblings?"*
Peter: *"Just a brother. We don't get along very well. I think that my parents understand him better than they understand me."*
BC: *"Is he somebody in your life now?"*
Peter: *"I feel that he is my brother now."*
BC: *"Do you have your own family? Wife, perhaps children?"*
Peter: *"No. There was a girl, but not anymore..."*
BC: *"What do you remember about her?"*
Peter: *"She was lovely. I liked her very much."*
BC: *"So what happened?"*

I waited for an answer, but nothing came out of Peter's mouth, so I instructed him to move to a scene that was relevant to what happened with the girl he had been in love with.

Peter: *"I am twenty now. There is that girl I really like. Her name is Rachel. I cannot marry her."*

BC: *"Why can you not?"*

Peter: *"Because of my parents."*

BC: *"How come?"*

There was a long pause until Peter answered. His tone was now sharp, even brutal.

Peter: *"It doesn't matter."*

BC: *"Can you be more specific?"*

When he answered, Peter's tone was louder He seemed irritated and angry.

Peter: *"I said it doesn't matter."*

I tried another time and I got the same answer. No matter how I formulated my questions, Peter kept telling me the same thing, louder and more aggressively, so I got the hint that he didn't want to recall more details or it was something he wasn't prepared to share, not even with me. I decided to distract his attention and ask a last question before I brought him back to complete awareness.

BC: *"What did you learn in the life you revisited?"*

Peter: *"Take instant decisions... decide on the spot."*

As the sun started going down, my practice room was filled in with all sorts of colors. The sky's shades were unbelievable. I felt peaceful while I waited for Peter to speak. When he did, he said that his memories from the past lives he revisited weren't a surprise for him. He said that in many ways his present life and the one of the farmer, living on a farm in England, had many similarities. I didn't want to intrude so I stopped asking questions, but I was sure that this time he knew that he had to make instant decisions.

I was stubborn enough to push him to share a little bit more. After a while, Peter admitted that he felt that, in the past life he revisited, his parents dominated his existence, demanding he acted according to their beliefs.

He vaguely recalled the reason for their involvement in his relationship with Rachel, the girl he remembered so well, and thought that something painful may have happened to her. Again, he didn't want to acknowledge what, but he was prepared to find out more about himself, because, before he left my practice, he booked in for another past life regression.

    In my opinion, there is a huge difference between a smart person and a wise one. One doesn't need to be highly clever to be wise. A smart person may have knowledge in several areas whilst a person with wisdom is one who acts on a very special gut feeling in making quick choices. You may have heard about business acumen, the ability to make fast decisions and change business strategies whenever it is required by specific circumstances. A wise person is one that can be characterized by this ability. Sometimes, opportunities come in the most unforeseen ways and in the most unexpected moments. One needs the capacity to make decisions on the spot; otherwise these possibilities would be wasted.

    Decisions have to be logical acts, separated from impulses. What I find interesting is that, in most cases, people take the opposite routes to the ones expected or instructed to do, not just because they rebel against domination or authority. People don't like to be told what to do. This is fair enough, because even if decisions are personal, the strategy behind them is common.

    When opportunity arises, we have to make sure it's worth it by examining what alternatives are available rather than by flipping a coin. However, we usually make heuristic choices, sometimes unnecessary, based on our perspective of the best alternative, which is currently available to us. These decisions may have roots in fatality, coincidence and randomness rather than in our own way of thinking and our individual problem-solving systems.

People say *"this won't work"* from time to time, but as a whole decision-making routine it fails to help us achieve success. However, even making random choices can have a mathematically formulated expectancy of error in information processing and cognitive quantum. *"Luck is what happens when preparation meets opportunity"*, as Seneca, the Roman Stoic Philosopher, once said.

Karmic lesson 20

CREATIVITY

"Put your heart into what you do"

Ella is one of those extraordinary women who has achieved success in every area of her life. In her mid fifties, she is a person with high class; she is also a very successful businesswoman and a good mother. She seems to have it all: career, personal life, great health and appealing appearance.

Ella is passionate about reading and her knowledge is immeasurable. I knew that I could build a strong rapport with her only if I was able to raise the conversation to her level. So, before asking details about her life, we firstly talked about books that changed our lives forever and we found that we had similar preferences. Then Ella started telling me about her children, which she brought up on her own after the break up of a marriage that still seemed painful for her. Ella was proud of her children's accomplishments, as every mother would be. She started her business while the children were still toddlers and was able to organize her life in a way that allowed both motherhood and career to work perfectly together.

I looked at her whilst she was talking about her present husband, a very special man who knew how to handle her, and all I was able to see was high class. She wore an immaculate light blue dress that complemented her blonde neck-length hair. The quality of her high-heel designer shoes and jewelry she wore gave me an idea of the financial independence she'd built for herself. My eyes caught a small amethyst brooch, in the shape of a flower, two vintage rings and a perfectly round sapphire pendant with fine watermarks. She looked pristine, calm and content.

I had regressed Ella a few times previously, so she knew what to expect. Therefore, I kept my induction and deepener short and a few minutes into it, Ella began sharing memories from one of her past lives.

Ella: *"I am in the Netherlands. I even remember my town. It starts with Alk..."*

Ella started spelling and there was no way of stopping her. It took her a few minutes until she pronounced the name of the town Alkmaar. Ella has never travelled to Holland.

BC: *"What do you remember about yourself?"*

Ella: *"I am a young woman of twenty-one. My hair is dark blonde; I wear it up. My skin is not pale, but not very dark either."*

BC: *"What are you wearing?"*

Ella: *"I wear a long green dress. It is tight on my waist and flows down to my ankles. I have a white collar with some little flower embroidery around my neck. It is quite cute. The fabric is not the softest, but it's warm."*

BC: *"Do you remember your name?"*

Ella: *"Anna. I believe that my name is longer than that, but everybody calls me Anna."*

BC: *"What about the year? Can you remember it?"*

Ella: *"1831."*

Ella was quite different to many of the people I knew, or at least in my opinion she was. Her answers came fast and were detailed, one after another, with that calmness specific to her.

BC: *"Remember now your happiest day in the lifetime as Anna."*

Ella: *"It's my wedding day. I am still twenty-one. I am in a small church outside of the town. I can hear the rain outside."*

BC: *"Who are you getting married to?"*

Ella: *"His name is Johan. He is twenty seven. He is taller than me, but not by much. Not a heavy built man... more like average build. He has short dark hair and olive skin. His eyes are blue."*

BC: *"Do you recognize him?"*

Ella kept silent for a moment and, while trying to remember, a fine line formed in between her eyebrows. Then she started crying quietly.

Ella: *"He is my husband now... same energy... same voice. He is so gentle and kind."*

BC: *"Are there many people at your wedding?"*

Ella: *"A few. I was born in a different part of the country. My parents are not here and I cannot remember why. I know that they are alive. Maybe it is too far for them to travel. Johan's mother is here... and a few friends."*

BC: *"Can you recognize any of them as being people you know in the present life?"*

Ella: *"Almost all of them... two are my friends now, one is my daughter now; the other one is my cousin. Amazing!"*

BC: *"What else can you remember from your weeding day?"*

Ella: *"I wear a white pretty dress with stripes of lace. It's beautiful really. Johan is so emotional. He has a soft heart."*

BC: *"Leave this memory now and go to another scene in that lifetime."*

Ella: *"I am in my house. Everything is spotless. There is a room at the back where I work."*

BC: *"What do you do?"*

Ella: *"I make tapestry. I have a big frame and all sorts of colored wool. Oh! I create beautiful things... carpets, rugs, blankets, art... Amazing things! Very well put together."*

BC: *"What does Johan do for living?"*

Ella: *"He works with his brother. They make cheese. Sometimes he helps me. I make good money. I sell everything and I even have orders. I see now... This is why we can afford beautiful things."*

BC: *"Tell me about your house."*

Ella: *"It's white with a kind of roof I've never seen before. White picket fence and a small garden at the front with beautiful flowers... all sorts of colors. There is a small kitchen... and a decorative plate with red apples painted on it on the wall. I love the kitchen! I believe that I love cooking too. In the living room, above the brown sofa, there is a painting of two cows. Oh! I think I made it. I am good with that!"*

BC: *"So what are you doing now?"*

Ella: *"Working. I make a blanket. It's greenish... like a landscape with a mountain, grass and some trees on it. It's beautiful. I look out the window for Johan. He has to come home for dinner. It smells like freshly baked bread. I see him now. He wears a black and grey sweater. He opens the gate. My heart is happy."*

BC: *"Do you love him?"*

Ella: *"Oh yes. He is so kind."*

Remembering the memory of her husband, Ella smiled and suddenly looked so much younger.

BC: *"Is it a happy life?"*

Ella: *"The happiest. My life is so peaceful."*

BC: *"Take me now to the worst memory in that lifetime."*

It took her a few minutes to answer. Tears started falling down her face, which she looked after so carefully.

Ella: *"I am in a small cemetery. It's raining. There is a hole in the ground and a casket at the bottom of it... It's Johan..."*

BC: *"What happened?"*

Ella: *"He died... young. He had a weak heart I guess and he just died. I am standing next to that hole and cry. I throw red flowers from my garden on the casket. It is raining on the casket and there is mud everywhere."*

BC: *"Are there any people around?"*

Ella: *"All his family and friends are here."*

BC: *"Do you recognize any of them?"*

Ella: *"They are all people I know now, friends, neighbors, cousins."*

BC: *"How old are you now?"*

Ella *"Twenty-four. I am devastated. His child will never know his father..."*

BC: *"Are you pregnant?"*

Ella: *"Yes, just five months pregnant."*

BC: *"Let this memory now fade away and remember the day when your child was born."*

Ella: *"It is daytime. I just gave birth to a baby boy... I am bleeding badly. I named my child Daniel. He is gorgeous. I hold him as I die!"*

I didn't expect that! What a sad life, I thought to myself, but Ella was of another opinion.

Ella: *"As I rise above my body, I look back on my life. I had the best man in the world. I loved him and he adored me. I had a beautiful home and I was able to make a living. And this boy... He is gorgeous."*

BC: *"Who will look after him?"*

Ella: *"One of Johan's brothers. They cannot have children. They will love him and take care of him!"*

BC: *"Do you recognize your son Daniel?"*
Ella: *"He is my son now."*
BC: *"Can you remember anything else from your life as Anna?"*
Ella: *"I am in the clouds. There is so much peace and love here. I am not sorry I died. I feel wonderful here. I hear somebody telling me that I am home. Oh! I can see Johan. He is smiling."*
BC: *"Do you remember what you were meant to achieve?"*
Ella: *"I learnt to be creative. I made the most beautiful things... art. Creativity... put your heart into what you do... make something from nothing!"*

After the session, we had a long talk. Ella was the last client of that day during a sunny March, so I had the time. She talked about creativity and the way she invented or perhaps reinvented herself when her first marriage fell apart. This woman had strength out of the ordinary, raising children on her own while creating a very successful business. For me, Ella was inspiring.

We usually associate creativity with art and artistry, when in fact this quality which few possess, points to originality in every aspect of our lives. It is true though that creativity refers to an ability to express ourselves, which in most cases is an art in itself. Art is part of our daily life and we understand it individually. However, Plato didn't believe in art. For him, a painter was just a crafter who mimicked reality. If he was correct, in the process of creativity, we may do exactly that: express in an authentic mode our own reality that may differ from others' perspectives. The final product is valuable if the point of view is original. This, in my opinion is what differentiates Pablo Picasso's innovative paintings from an abstract scribbler.

For me, creativity mostly describes an original vision that may inspire others. I believe that inventiveness discloses the potential to adapt and change strategies when required, using the ability of imagination and unconformity. I refer to original ideas versus a new way of putting them into action. An unorthodox way of thinking, based on the fact that whatever the mind sees can be reproduced, or brought to life in reality, this, for me, is a creative one; the act of creation itself being based on structure mapping and analogies.

Those close to the business field may have heard about the four *"P"* in the equation of creativity. They refer to a *"person"*, in a certain *"place"*, who can create a *"product"*, designed in a specific *"process"*. In day-to-day life, we follow the same order in designing our own life as an authentic masterpiece. Our lives are in fact blank canvases, which we express ourselves on, as long as we breathe in and out.

Karmic lesson 21

SOLITUDE

"People are important"

Vivian has one of those personalities that would never go unnoticed. She is wise, always has a good word to say and a shoulder to lean on for the one who needs it. Vivian is a teacher and I am sure that her little students are blessed to know her. She is in her forties, but has already impacted so many lives so far.

I met her on one occasion right after she moved to my town and my first impression was that she was absolutely awesome. I was therefore delighted when she booked in for a past life regression. She arrived one Monday evening, straight from work and she seemed fresh like she'd come from an afternoon nap. She was full of energy, and enthusiasm was written all over her face.

We talked for a little while and she admitted that she noticed some patterns in her life that kept repeating, and thought that she may have carried something from a past life that was triggering recurring events in the present. As she talked, I observed her beautiful brown eyes that complemented her olive skin. Vivian looked majestic and exotic. She was truly a beautiful woman with a lovely personality. She wasn't shy and she wasn't too out there. She was polite and sure about herself.

Once ready to start, Vivian relaxed and very soon answered my questions.

Vivian: *"I am a little girl. I wear rags... like a sack. I am barefoot, but my feet are pale and clean. My hair is short and brown... my eyes blue."*

BC: *"How old are you?"*

Vivian: *"I am maybe seven years old."*

BC: *"What do you see when you look around? Are you indoors or outdoors?"*

Vivian: *"I see nature. I am outdoors... just standing outside. It is quiet. I feel like I'm lost and I don't know the way back home. I was following nature and I got lost."*

BC: *"What do you remember about your home?"*

Vivian: *"It's like a cabin... very small... somewhere in England. I live with my parents."*

BC: *"What do you remember about them?"*

Vivian: *"Hmm... they are never around. They work hard... on the land."*

BC: *"What is your name?"*

Vivian: *"My name is Sarah."*

BC: *"I want you now to go to another moment as Sarah."*

Vivian: *"I am thirteen now. I am at home alone. My parents are working."*

BC: *"Look around and tell me what you see."*

Vivian: *"It's tidy, but small. The cabin is surrounded by trees... very tall trees."*

BC: *"Now focus on your mother. What can you remember about her?"*

Vivian: *"Her name is Ruth. She is tired... working too hard."*

BC: *"Can you recognize her energy?"*

Vivian: *"Yes. She is my friend."*

She started smiling whilst naming her best friend in the present. Vivian looked even more appealing as she smiled.

BC: *"Now focus on your father and tell me what you remember about him."*

Vivian: *"He is the same father I have today. I am scared of him."*

BC: *"Why is that?"*

Vivian: *"He drinks too much. He seems big and dark. He is scary."*

BC: *"Do you remember the year?"*

Vivian: *"It's 1672."*

BC: *"Leave this scene behind and move to another one."*

Vivian: *"I am alone again. I wear a long dress with an apron. My parents are gone... they died a while back."*

BC: *"How old are you now?"*

Vivian: *"Not quite thirty."*

BC: *"Do you live in the same cabin?"*

Vivian: *"Yes, working the land like my parents did. Nobody around..."*

BC: *"So no partner in your life..."*

Vivian: *"No. I have the feeling that I live too far away from people. The cabin is too far away from everybody."*

BC: *"Don't worry about that. Move now to another moment in the lifetime as Sarah."*

Vivian: *"I am in the same place. I am old and still alone. I am ready to die. I die of old age."*

BC: *"So you are still alone..."*

Vivian: *"I was never able to find a man... any man... or friends. Very sad life!"*

BC: *"Experience now the moment of your soul leaving the body and, as you do that, remember what you learnt in that lifetime."*

Vivian: *"Solitude... There was no one to trust..."*

As she remembered the main lesson for the life as Sarah, Vivian seemed sad and there was no wonder why. She remembered a life lived in complete isolation, far away from people. I thought that it was fair to have another try, so I instructed her to recall another lifetime. I just hoped that it might have been a happier one.

Vivian: *"I am in a city. I want to say that I am in New York. I am a man, wearing business work shoes and a suit... just an average suit, not an expensive one."*

BC: *"Tell me about your work. Can you remember what work you do?"*

Vivian: *"Office work in a big office, surrounded by tall buildings. There are many other people in the same office."*

BC: *"What year is it?"*

Vivian: *"Mid 1900s."*

BC: *"How old are you?"*

Vivian: *"I am thirty-two."*

BC: *"Do you remember your name?"*

Vivian: *"Steven."*

BC: *"Do your have a family of your own; maybe a wife or children?"*

Vivian: *"I have a wife and a baby. My wife's name is Sarah. She is young and pretty. I am happy with her. The baby is a girl."*

BC: *"Do you recognize any of their energies?"*

Vivian: *"Not my wife's. My little baby is my granddaughter now."*

BC: *"So what are you doing on that street?"*

Vivian: *"I am going to work. As I get there, I can see my office. It is a huge room with many people. Everybody works in the same room."*

BC: *"That is great. Leave now this scene and move to another one."*

Vivian: *"I am in a town. It's sunny. I moved out from the city. I bought a house in this town. I feel happy here."*

BC: *"Is your family with you?"*

Vivian: *"Yes. We are all happy. My wife loves it here. My daughter is seven now."*

BC: *"Are you still working in the city?"*

Vivian: *"I do the same job, but not in the city."*

BC: *"I want you now to remember the happiest moment in that lifetime."*

Vivian: *"My daughter is getting married to a nice guy. She is happy so I am happy. I feel sad though that I am going to lose her, but she doesn't live far away."*

BC: *"What else do you remember?"*

Vivian: *"Sarah is wearing a pretty dress... a blue dress. It suits her."*

BC: *"Now go the last moments in that lifetime."*

Vivian: *"I am seventy-eight. I am in a hospital, wearing pajamas."*

BC: *"Why are you in the hospital?"*

Vivian: *"Lungs..."*

BC: *"Do you see any people around?"*

Vivian: *"My family is with me. They are sad."*

BC: *"Was it a happy or a sad life?"*

Vivian: *"Neither... just busy working and living."*

BC: *"How do you mean?"*

Vivian: *"I wished I didn't have my walls up. Besides my family, I was quite a loner."*

BC: *"Is there any residual energy you carried into the present?"*

Vivian: *"Yes. I was often alone. I carried that with me."*

As Vivian spoke, I looked at my shiny clock on the wall and remembered that I bought it more than a year ago. I fell in love with it when I first saw it on a website and couldn't resist. So I bought it and waited around six weeks for it to arrive. Then it took me another few days to put it together and stick the shiny numbers on the wall. It ended up covering a circle of more than a meter in diameter. So I admired it again and, realizing that there was enough time for one more life. I thought to myself, let's hope Vivian is third time lucky, remembering perhaps a happier life.

Vivian: *"I am a three year old girl. I wear a blue dress and seem very happy, laughing... very happy indeed. I am in a house with my parents around."*

BC: *"Do you recognize any of their energies as being people you know in the present life?"*

Vivian: *"My mother is my mother now. She is a happy woman. She loves me."*

BC: *"What is your name?"*

I noticed that Vivian was trying to remember her name. I thought that she couldn't because her first memories from the lifetime she revisited were of a three year old girl. But I was wrong.

Vivian: *"Yvonne is my name."*

BC: *"Great. If there is nothing else you can remember, go now to a relevant scene in the same lifetime."*

Vivian: *"I am married now to a good man. He is my husband in the present... same person."*

BC: *"Do you remember the year?"*

Vivian: *"1618."*

BC: *"How is the place you and your husband live?"*

Vivian: *"We don't have a home. We are travelling. I have been everywhere. We are young and exploring. My husband works here and there as we travel. He goes to homes and works for people and makes money. Now we are in Spain."*

BC: *"Brilliant. What else can you remember from the same lifetime?"*

Vivian: *"I am fifty now. We have children and grandchildren. Everybody is kind; nobody is hurting... close family."*

BC: *"Do you recognize any of them?"*

Vivian: *"All of them. They are exactly the children I have now."*

BC: *"Anything else?"*

Vivian: *"I lost one of my sons. He died in a sort of accident. I am devastated."*

BC: *"Now going further in time, do you remember who passed away first, your husband or you?"*

Vivian: *"My husband did. He just went a few days ago... I am old now... My children would have to take care of me somehow. One of them would look after me for sure..."*

BC: *"What about you? Do you remember how you passed?"*

Vivian: *"I am in my home. I don't want to live anymore. I am too old to. I am happy to go."*

BC: *"Do you remember what the lesson was for the lifetime you revisited?"*

Vivian: *"Don't live alone. People are important... family is important."*

BC: *"Is there any energy you carry into the present?"*

Yvonne: *"I felt alone after my husband passed... sad about being alone... deeply alone."*

Right after she opened her eyes, Vivian started talking again. I already knew that she loved people and was surrounded by family and friends, so, revisiting lives when she felt lonely was quite surprising, but perhaps necessary for her soul's journey. But again, the expectations of a regression don't always meet reality.

Being in your own company can be rewarding, but to achieve such contentment you have to be your own best friend. Therefore, for me, solitude is a state of finding myself rather than feeling alone. We falsely associate solitude with isolation, when in fact the inner peace created in a phase of temporary solitude has nothing to do with living as a troglodyte. Just remember the self-awareness of someone who can exclude themselves from the exterior world that surrounds them and ultimately surrender to the Universe itself. This contemplative state can be achieved in meditation.

    I taught meditation for a while and I know that introspection is not an easy task to learn; one needs time and practice to reach that supreme state I call 'musing', or finding inspiration from within. I would mention for those who have never practiced it that meditation finds its etymology in the Latin *"meditare"* that refers to thinking or contemplating. Whilst Western society may have a different approach to mindfulness, *"Dhyana"* is a primordial act of self-transcending in Hinduism and Buddhism. For Jainism, *"Ratnatraya"*, also referred to as *"Three Jewels"* is associated with aiming for salvation; the *"jewels"* to achieve it are conduct, knowledge and faith. For Taoism, creation and growth of vital energy force called *"qi"* can be achieved through meditation. If for Judaism, contemplation was a practice based on the Torah, which is the main spiritual book for this religion, for Christianity, personal devotion is mainly associated with prayer.

    Our Western world has grabbed little bits from all of these main beliefs where meditation was a common practice, and formed a comfortable amalgam of finding inner peace. A modern practice of yoga usually accompanies these practices. There is nothing wrong with this; whatever works for one in order to clear stress out and find inner peace is acceptable. However I would argue that many so called *"gurus"* who initiated small groups promised self-contentment took advantage of so many. In reality, things are so simple: if you want peace and harmony, all you have to do is to start that inner conversation with yourself. In solitude, listen and find the right answers!

Karmic lesson 22

TEMPTATION

"Be in control"

I try not to book appointments for the weekends, and when I got a phone call from my client Claire who asked me to fit her daughter in, my initial thought was no way. But she was insistent and explained that her daughter Jessica was visiting from Sydney, Australia and going back on Monday. So, as a favor to her mother, I booked her in.

I woke up that Saturday morning and wondered whether or not this would create a precedent. People talk and, once you make an amendment to your own schedule, many want to take advantage of it.

Jessica arrived right on time and while we had the initial talk, I observed her. She was exactly what I thought a corporate person these days would look like. I expected her to wear casual clothes because it was very early on a weekend day. Instead, she wore a pristine white shirt, pencil black skirt and black high heels. Her full make up was immaculate too. She wore her dark blonde hair up in a perfect hairdo and I had to remind myself that there was no hairdressing salon open at eight o'clock on a Saturday morning. Skinny, toned and oozing health, Jessica had fitness written all over her body.

So we talked and she explained that she had an obsession with her body. At first I didn't understand, but then she elaborated on the various diets she had been on for her whole life and the long hours she spent every day in a fitness centre. For Jessica, everything was about appearance and to keep herself in perfect shape, she even went through some plastic surgery procedures. Jessica was married to a man who seemed to be her perfect clone; same worries about how he looked, same high paid corporate job. They were happy, Jessica told me, and a child wouldn't have fitted into their perfect family. So they decided right after they got married 15 years ago, not to extend their family.

Jessica heard about past life regressions and, back in Sydney, she even met a hypnosis therapist, but never had the confidence to do a regression herself. But now, when her mother mentioned her memories in past lives, she decided to give it a try. So, I started the procedure of relaxing her and a few minutes later she shared her own memories coming from a very distant past.

Jessica: *"I am a woman... a tall, beautiful young woman."*

BC: *"What do you wear?"*

Jessica: *"A red below-the-knee dress and a white apron."*

BC: *"What else do you remember about yourself?"*

Jessica: *"I am twenty-five years old. Beautiful woman... dark hair, green eyes."*

BC: *"What is your name?"*

Jessica: *"My name is Clara."*

BC: *"Now look around and tell me what you see."*

Jessica: *"It's a bakery... yes, I am in a bakery... baking cakes... it's my bakery in the middle of a town in France... not Paris... another town."*

BC: *"Is there anything else that catches your attention?"*

Jessica: *"There are cakes everywhere. It's early in the morning... no clients yet. I believe that I am successful."*

I had the feeling that I caught a glimpse of pride on Jessica's face when she mentioned success.

BC: *"Can you remember the year?"*

Jessica: *"It's... hmm... 1893."*

I instructed her to go to another moment in time, perhaps one when she was in her own home.

Jessica: *"I own a little house with roses in the front garden. I am married to a man called Claude. He is young and happy... blue eyes, blonde hair, white skin... We are very much in love."*

BC: *"Can you recognize his energy?"*

Jessica: *"He is my father now."*

BC: *"What does he do for a living?"*

Jessica: *"I believe that he is a butcher and owns a little shop next to the bakery."*

BC: *"Do you have children?"*

Jessica: *"I don't believe we can. We tried, but..."*

BC: *"Remember now another memory from the same lifetime as I count from one to three."*

I started counting, still noticing Jessica's reactions. She looked like she was going through a lot of emotions. To be perfectly honest, it may have been the first time when she was letting her feelings show.

Jessica: *"I may be thirty now. I am baking a wedding cake for my friend. She is getting married tomorrow. I decorate it with yellow roses."*

BC: *"Anything else?"*

Jessica: *"I started being rounder. I cannot say 'no' to sweets. I am still beautiful... just curvier."*

That may have come as a surprise for her, as this woman was almost perfect and to let herself go with the flow would have been a shock.

BC: *"You have a sweet tooth..."*

Jessica: *"I think so... I taste everything and, when I finish work, I have a few slices of cakes."*

BC: *"And how is Claude doing?"*

Jessica: *"I feel that he is not so interested in me anymore... he is not looking at me as he did."*

Jessica couldn't remember what might have changed her husband's behavior towards her. After asking a few times without any specific response, I decided to move forward with the session.

BC: *"That's fine. Move now in time to a significant memory"*

Jessica: *"I am at home waiting for Claude. It's late and he is still not home."*

BC: *"How old are you now?"*

Jessica: *"Maybe thirty-five or thirty-six. I wear a nightgown... Dear me... I am fat... The cakes made me gain that weight."*

BC: *"Don't worry about that. So what happens?"*

Jessica kept silent for a very long time. Her perfect body looked so small and helpless on the recliner.

Jessica: *"I think that Claude left me for my neighbor. I heard that something was going on, but never believed it."*

BC: *"Do you recognize her?"*

Jessica: *"Yes, she is my best friend now."*

BC: *"So he left you..."*

Jessica: *"Yes. They moved to another town... I don't know where. They just disappeared... I had to close down the butchery."*

I guided her to another scene and she started talking straight away. This time she seemed happier.

Jessica: *"I may be just over forty now. My bakery is a success... I am a success."*

BC: *"How do you mean?"*

Jessica: *"I am beautiful again... lost the weight... starved myself... I learnt how to manage my addiction to sugar."*

BC: *"Are you happy?"*

Jessica: *"Very happy indeed."*

BC: *"Have you heard from Claude?"*

Jessica: *"Not from him. A customer told me that she had seen them. They are not happy... they are miserable. She cannot have children either... Oh well..."*

BC: *"Any other man in the horizon?"*

Jessica: *"I don't want another one. I am happy on my own. I have a good life. I have many friends and love my life as it is."*

BC: *"Go now to the last moments in that lifetime and, when you are in the scene, tell me what you see."*

Jessica: *"I am old... maybe around ninety. I am in a kind of old people's home... like a retirement home. It's very nice here. I believe that I die of old age... very peaceful..."*

BC: *"What did you learn as Clara?"*

Jessica: *"Addiction... temptation. Be in control... don't give in to anything!"*

Jessica opened her eyes and took a minute to compose herself. Looking at her, I saw that this beautiful woman understood exactly why her subconscious decided to revisit the life she did. We kept talking for a few minutes before she left and as she walked towards her car, I couldn't stop admiring her beauty and perfect posture.

Jessica keeps in touch and at least once a week she drops me an email or a text message, and anytime I get a sign from her, I notice how much more relaxed she is. Her point of view on beauty in general might have started to change after the regression.

We refer to temptations as guilty pleasures, usually highlighting a side to ourselves we cannot control. Some may have the self-discipline to resist them; others may lack confidence and power and surrender to addictions entering their lives. Many people point out alcohol, smoking and drugs as the main temptations - and therefore addictions - forgetting that every obsession could start dependence. We may be addicted to everything money can buy, or to seeing reality distorted through lies and cheating, for instance, without actually being compulsory liars. Some can even be obsessed with other people, therefore not able to move forward in life without having them around.

To be perfectly honest, these days there are so many temptations. Even if some may be in the grey area or under the religious umbrella, everything that could represent a possible blandishment is a forbidden sin; and avoiding it is a matter of choice. Sin for Christianity is replicated in Buddhism as the demon Mara who tempted the prince Siddhartha, the Buddha. According to the legend, whilst he was in a meditation state, Mara's daughters tried seducing him without any success. Exactly as in other religions, he had made the choice of continuing his enlightenment and not giving in to the visions. What Christianity, for instance, defines as sin, Buddhism describes as *"Raga"* or desire.

Unfortunately, we are tempted because we perceive a short-term reward in everything that may produce a state of instant pleasure or enjoyment at a moment in time. I am sure that we would be surprised to discover how a computer game, social media use and the Internet in general could raise our endorphins. They may be all necessary, as long as they don't take over our lives.

The answer to resisting temptation, in my opinion, is knowing what we actually need and what we can't live without, and perhaps understanding that the adventure and adrenaline rush temptations' cause is just an illusion.

BRIGITTE CALLOWAY

Karmic lesson 23

RESPECT

"Consider other people's feelings"

When the phone rang, the voice at the other end was strong and I sensed a Latino accent that I totally loved. The man introduced himself as Mateo and asked for the next available appointment. When I offered him a booking for Friday morning in two weeks' time, he tried negotiating for an earlier date, but since I couldn't accommodate him any earlier, he had to settle for what I suggested initially.

He arrived on that Friday morning and, as I opened the door, I knew that this was a man of not many words. I looked at him walking down the corridor and noticed that he was quite handsome. Maybe in his late forties, Mateo was dark, slim, fit and quite elegant in his cream colored pants and black shirt.

When he started talking with that strong voice, he seemed opinionated and strong willed. He cut me off a few times and I thought to myself that this session would turn into a fiasco if I didn't handle it well. So I listened to everything he said about himself, knowing that my forte was to use every detail he shared in creating the necessary rapport between us.

Mateo left his Hispanic country five years ago and embarked on a trip to New Zealand where he got a well-paid contract in the oil industry. His wife and daughter followed him. He liked his new country, but said that it may be just a temporary destination because his wife wasn't able to settle properly. From what he said, I understood that he and his seven year old daughter would have loved to live here forever, but his wife missed her family, friends and the sense of belonging in general their birth country gave her. Therefore, Mateo knew that he may have to follow her back or say goodbye to his marriage. At this stage however, he constantly fought with his wife and thought that he may be able to change her mind. He battled to stay whilst she defended herself and demanded to go.

Under the mask of power and strength, Mateo was quite sensitive and when he mentioned a few phobias he'd accumulated in the last few years, I offered a traditional hypnotherapy cure, but he knew better. He wanted a past life regression and was firm in his beliefs that none of his fears would have had roots in the present. He was even inclined to believe that nobody on this planet could hypnotize him, but was prepared to give it a try, maybe just to prove to me that he was right. I wouldn't be the one to contradict him, so I made sure that he felt comfortable in the recliner, checked the room temperature and started the session. Outside, it was hot and sticky.

A good half an hour later, Mateo started answering my questions, this time with a very soft voice, and I thought to myself that this strong man was just about to have the revelation of his life as he was in that deep hypnosis state he didn't believe in initially.

Mateo: *"I am a young man of maybe twenty-three. I have curly blonde hair and very white skin... longer hair, down to my shoulders... and blue eyes. "*

BC: *"Do you remember your name?"*

Mateo: *"Samuel."*

BC: *"What can you see when you look around?"*

Mateo: *"I am outdoors... somewhere on a street in Italy... maybe in Rome... walking. There is rock everywhere... looks like the road is paved with rocks."*

BC: *"What year it is?"*

Mateo: *"I think it's 1692."*

BC: *"Do you have any family?"*

Mateo: *"I am the youngest of eleven... ten sisters before me. My parents have a small textile manufacturer... I think that they dye fabric... they are doing well..."*

BC: *"Tell me about your sisters."*

Mateo: *"They are all married... some have children... many nephews and nieces... I am not married..."*

BC: *"Why are you not married?"*

Mateo: *"Hmm..."*

Mateo's face changed suddenly and I had the feeling that he was trying to hide something rather than not remembering, so I reformulated my question.

BC: *"Do you have a lover?"*

Mateo: *"I love somebody, but nobody knows... not even her."*

BC: *"Who is she?"*

Mateo: *"The woman I love... Elena ... she is married to my best friend Nardo... and has children. She doesn't know..."*

BC: *"Have you tried telling her?"*

Mateo: *"I respect her too much. She loves her husband... I believe that she loves me too, but she cannot* do anything about it...or about us... Nardo is my best friend!"

Mateo seemed sad and I sympathized with the man he was in a past life, who couldn't share his feelings with a married woman.

BC: *"Is Elena somebody you know in the present?"*

Mateo: *"Hmmm... my wife now. She is my wife! Yes, she is!"*

BC: *"What about your sisters? Can you recognize any of them?"*

Mateo: *"The eldest is my daughter and another one is my brother. I think that there is another sister I know... yes, she is my cousin now."*

BC: *"What about your parents?"*

Mateo: *"My mother is my mother now... my father seems familiar too... but I don't know who he is..."*

I instructed him to move a few years later in time and waited for a while until he spoke again. To be perfectly honest, I was curious to hear if his love was reciprocated.

Mateo: *"I am forty now. My parents are not alive anymore and I run the manufacturing business... I live in their old house..."*

BC: *"Tell me about Elena."*

Mateo: *"We are friends... she is my best friend's wife... She doesn't know I have feelings for her... my mother knew before she died, but she never raised the subject..."*

BC: *"Do you think that she would want to know?"*

Mateo: *"She cannot do anything about it! Her husband is a good man and she loves him... they have two sons together."*

BC: *"Is her husband Nardo somebody you know?"*

Mateo: *"My father... and one of his sons is my brother-in-law."*

Mateo moved another few years in time without being instructed, so I let him remember what he wanted to.

Mateo: *"I am sixty-two now. Elena is sick... very sick. She coughs blood... I visit her family everyday!"*

BC: *"Is Nardo still alive?"*

Mateo: *"Yes, he is. I feel sorry for him. He is a good man."*

BC: *"Go on..."*

Mateo: *"I think that Elena is dying... yes, she is. I look into her eyes and I know that she knows I love her... she loves me too... her eyes are telling me that... but I respect her too much to create problems..."*

BC: *"So she is dying..."*

Mateo: *"Now!"*

Tears started flowing down on his face and his voice got even softer. He suffered, I knew that much!

BC: *"Don't worry too much. There is nothing you can do. Maybe move a few years later and tell me what you see."*

Mateo: *"I am sixty-five now... Every night I cry after Elena... she is long gone."*

BC: *"And her husband?"*

Mateo: *"I go every day and visit him... and help with money... he doesn't know anything. He married another woman... she is nice..."*

BC: *"You are a good friend. I want you now to remember the moment you died."*

Mateo: *"I am older... maybe almost seventy. There is something bad with my back... like it's broken or something... something hit me or I fell... I cannot remember... I just die on the street."*

BC: *"What else can you remember from the lifetime as Samuel?"*

Mateo: *"I go where Elena is. I don't see her, but I feel her presence... I am happy. I look down and I see her children. I left them everything I owned... they are sorted."*

BC: *"What was your lesson as Samuel?"*

Mateo: *"Respect... consider other people's feelings... I have done very well! Elena is proud of me... angels are proud of me..."*

I gave Mateo a few minutes before I asked him to return to complete awareness. He opened his eyes and looked straight into mine. He wasn't confused at all and the first thought that came to my mind was that this man's life may have changed forever. Recalling memories from a past life can have a strong impact on everybody and he was no different.

After asking what his feelings were about the lifetime he revisited, I let him talk for a while without interrupting him. *"My wife and I should make a compromise"*, he said, hoping that the future would make one of them change their minds with regards to going back to their birth country, or living in New Zealand forever. From the position of a warrior he became a negotiator, I thought to myself, whilst looking at the steamy window. I realized that the humidity outside will have been very high. There were no signs of rain and I knew that outside it might have felt like being in a sauna.

The first time I heard from Mateo after his regression was at the end of last year. He emailed to let me know that his wife got a job in the hospitality industry and felt more at peace with her life. He also said that he booked a trip back to Spain a few months from then, first trip in five years, and that he had bought himself some time until their final decision, just by respecting the fact that his wife wanted to see her people. The second time he emailed me was last week. He was in Spain and seemed in good spirits. *"We are having a great holiday. Now it's time to come back home"*, he wrote. I smiled reading his email remembering what a drop of respect can do in one's life!

We respect people who matter to us; we look up to their actions or reactions, which have certain significance for us. We cherish and we ask to be appreciated, sometimes ignoring the fact that, in order to be recognized, we first need to respect ourselves. Our lack of self-esteem stops us from achieving goals and making ourselves noticed. Nobody would consider us if we don't first! Confucius once said *"Respect yourself and others will respect you"*. Over two thousand years later, his saying is still applicable.

The whole of society should be based on respect and the lack of it in relationships is visible these days. We tend to forget about politeness and courtesy in many situations and we seem to blame our lack of respect on other people's behavior. Respect has nothing to do with veneration though and not with humbleness either: we don't have to put our heads down, kiss somebody's feet or praise people.

In the culture I was born in, people still use *"servus"* as a form of salutation. The term has its roots in the Latin *"servus hummilius"* that means *"at your service"*, therefore from a young age I understood that tolerance, acceptance and courtesy are in general what respect is based on. Each culture though has its own acceptable etiquette with regards to respect and disrespect. In some societies, looking or not looking into somebody's eyes, touching people's hands or feet or using certain words are forms of disrespect. There is however a common acceptance of a concept of behavior, which shows respect for our fellow humans, and that is based on acting as we wish others to act to us.

EPILOGUE

"My soul is from elsewhere, I am sure of that, and I intend to end up there"

Rumi

I started writing this book a while back in New Zealand and struggled to find the time to put together the cases I intended to present in it. My hypnotherapy practice was my priority and my hectic work life didn't allow too much time for writing.

I finished the book in Bali, where for a period of time I rekindled myself; I witnessed Hindu practices, I talked with people about their beliefs and I was lucky enough to meet people who believed in karma and reincarnation. I looked at the magnificent temples and tried to grasp as many details as I was able to. In Bali, I realized that I was not the only one who believed in reincarnating all over again with people we know now. My ideas were common practice there and that gave me a certain peace, necessary to finish my book.

Still in Bali, I decided that the number of karmic case studies I put together for my readers are enough to give a good understanding that there are many things we have to learn through each incarnation. There may be many more too; maybe hundreds, maybe thousands, maybe millions... who knows... With each achievement, we become better, more open and tolerant to other people's needs and definitely more loving. With every assignment, we identify the similarity with other fellow humans. We are all the same. We are all on the road to success, learning, growing and evolving with each life we live.

I am sure that there are many people who are skeptical of the whole idea of past life regression under hypnosis. Some may even believe in reincarnation but cannot accept that now, in this very moment in time that somebody could help them remember aspects from other lives they have lived before. To them I would say that it is not the hypnotist who has the answers; it is their own subconscious mind that recalls the memories, because the therapist's only role is to induce hypnosis and ask questions.

I am also positive that some will find it hard to believe that their mothers now, for instance, may have been their spouses in other lives. It is not a straightforward concept, I agree. But it is as it is. I can assure you that most of my clients may have been in your shoes before regressing and remembering memories from past lives. They changed their minds after though.

To all the people who still have doubts regarding the concept of past life regression, I would say that sometimes we believe in things we see and other times in the things we don't. Do whatever works for you, believe or not, but my advice would be to keep an open heart until you experience a regression for yourself to a past existence, and perhaps make your mind up after.

And lastly, I would like to address the people who find it hard to recover after losing beloved ones. It is not the first time you have lived with them and it won't be the last time you see them either. They will come back to you in another existence! Don't lose hope and don't live in sadness. You have an assignment to achieve now, exactly as they did before they left you. It is never forever!

Finishing my book in Bali was the best thing I could have done. As I was sitting on the esplanade, I realized that we are all particles of sand forming a wide beach; none of us more important than others, no matter at what stage of evolvement we may be. Some may be washed away by waves; others stay dry on the beach. For centuries, with each low and high tide and with each wave, all the particles get reunited on the beach. We, humans, are the same; with each reincarnation, we come back into each other's lives.

BRIGITTE CALLOWAY

ABOUT THE AUTHOR

Brigitte Calloway is a hypnotherapist, who lives and maintains a private practice in Inglewood, New Zealand. She practices traditional hypnotherapy as well as past life regression hypnosis. Her first book "You have lived many times" was published in 2018.

www.ingramcontent.com/pod-product-compliance
Lightning Source LLC
Chambersburg PA
CBHW071353290426
44108CB00014B/1529